YOU CAN COPE WITH

Peripheral Neuropathy

365 Tips for Living a Better Life

YOU CAN COPE WITH
Peripheral Neuropathy

365 Tips for Living a Better Life

Mims Cushing
Norman Latov, MD, PhD

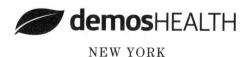

demosHEALTH

NEW YORK

Visit our web site at www.demosmedpub.com

Library of Congress Cataloging-in-Publication Data

Cushing, Mims.
  You can cope with peripheral neuropathy : 365 tips for living a better life / Mims Cushing, Norman Latov.
    p. cm.
  Includes bibliographical references and index.
  ISBN 978-1-932603-76-7
  1. Nerves, Peripheral—Diseases—Popular works.   I. Latov, Norman.   II. Title.
  RC409.C87 2009
  616.8—dc22   2009006939

Special discounts on bulk quantities of Demos Health books are available to corporations, professional associations, pharmaceutical companies, health care organizations, and other qualifying groups. For details, please contact:

Special Sales Department
Demos Medical Publishing
11 W. 42nd Street, 15th Floor
New York, NY 10036
Phone: 800–532–8663 or 212–683–0072
Fax: 212–941–7842
www.demoshealth.com

Made in the United States of America

09 10 11 12   5 4 3

Contents

     Norman Latov

11. Frequently Asked Questions   139
     Norman Latov

12. The Hope of Research   147
     Norman Latov

13. Peripheral Neuropathy Stories by Those Who Know It Best   151
     Mims Cushing

     The Neuropathy Association's Designated Neuropathy Centers   *183*

     Resources   *185*

     Acronyms   *191*

     Bibliography   *193*

     Index   *199*

Preface

Be careful about reading health books. You may die of a misprint.
—Mark Twain

When I was in school, back in the 1950s, from third grade through twelfth, everyone was required to take athletics, Monday through Friday. How I loved getting out of sports. Mother wouldn't give me a "Sports Excuse" very often, so I had to run in field hockey, lacrosse, basketball. In winter, we had the dreaded running races in the gym. But I did like to walk. My Mom and I went into New York City from Larchmont on weekends and traipsed up and down Madison or Fifth Avenues at a breakneck pace. I didn't have neuropathy. Yet.

Feet to Brain: Are You There?

When we moved to Ponte Vedra Beach, Florida, in 1991, I enjoyed walking to Lakeside, a community near mine; however, in 1996, people passed me by and soon were far ahead. My 30-minute walk took 40 minutes. Friends wanted me to go faster, but my feet didn't like the idea. My legs were losing strength, a common problem with neuropathy. My feet were tingling, burning, and numb—especially at night. I felt stabbing, shooting pains. Ding. Ding. Ding. Bells and whistles should have sounded an alarm, but they didn't. In the 1990s, few people knew about peripheral neuropathy, myself included. A huge number still haven't a clue about it, even though 20 million people in the United States have peripheral neuropathy. And the numbers are growing.

In 1996, I went to an internist because the symptoms made me crabby. She said, "You may have peripheral neuropathy. See a neurologist." Her quick diagnosis was unusual. Not so long ago, some patients weren't diagnosed for a long time. Thirty-four years is the longest I've heard of.

Your neuropathy may not involve the feet. It can involve any part of the body associated with the peripheral nervous system, although a neurologist at the University of Florida & Shands Jacksonville told me that 75% of his practice revolves around foot problems.

I procrastinated, then a few months later had blood tests, which resulted in no conclusions. That's often the case with early neuropathy, because nerves don't show the damage on tests until well after symptoms begin. Many years later, I had electromyography tests, which show the effects of the nerves on the muscles and sometimes give doctors a lot of information; but not in my case.

I forged ahead, ignoring daytime symptoms. At night I tossed in bed, trying to figure out how to sleep without the top sheet driving my feet crazy. Nights meant nightmares, days meant daymares.

By autumn of 1999, something had to be done. That Thanksgiving, I tried to wear pretty shoes, not even killer spikes. I couldn't wait for the day to be over. Later that evening at home, I discovered The Neuropathy Association website. Sitting in the kitchen, looking at my monitor, I felt tears running relay races down my cheeks. I was happy to know I wasn't dreaming up the whole issue, grateful to find I wasn't crazy, although stunned to realize the symptoms were not going to disappear, according to the Internet.

I could wait no longer. I found a doctor who listened and cared. After arranging for me to have a blood workup and quantitative sensory testing, he told me I probably had sensory neuropathy, cause unknown. He said further results of the blood tests would most likely confirm his initial diagnosis. It did. He gave me a prescription to try to control the burning, tingling, and numbness.

Senior Moments Turn into Senior Months

The meds helped ease the burning, but for me the side effects were nasty. I felt decades older than my age of 55. My short-term memory was shot, and I had to take naps, morning and afternoon. I'd fall asleep in movies or at a symphony or lecture.

Once, at a play, I must have been snoring. I was in the front row and awoke with a jolt and a loud snort, with all the actors looking at me. Some days, I barely made it through my 2-hour writers' roundtable sessions. As people read their stories, I put one hand on my forehead, bent my head down, and catnapped. When teaching writing classes, I couldn't remember what I'd said 5 minutes before. When I taped a class, I was horrified at my redundancies. I had to be super-organized and write everything down in the order in which I wanted to say it. I wish I'd known my memory problems would end once I kicked the drug.

After a few years, I weaned myself off the meds, following the doctor's instructions. My intense fatigue lessened, and today my memory issues are the same as the rest of my furry-brained, 60-plus friends.

Maybe I'm less annoyed by the symptoms because I've given strict instructions to my brain to stop whining. Peripheral neuropathy for me means lousy days, followed by great ones. But sometimes perfect mornings can turn into afternoons that belong in the garbage.

Alice Had the Answer

If you asked my Aunt Alice, who died at 101 and was no taller than a doorknob, "How are you?" she might say, "Oh, I have pneumonia, but I am not giving it the respect it wants." In her 90s, with bad arthritis, she still drove "the old people" to Catholic Mass.

I love her attitude. If somebody says, "How are you?" I say, "Fine!" Because if I am out and about, then I am fine. If *I* don't want to hear about *my* pains, why should anyone else? I'm not lying; it simply makes me feel better to say "I'm fine." Why tell people, "Yesterday stunk. I could barely walk from the parking lot to Publix."

I read somewhere that people with peripheral neuropathy might qualify for a handicap placard, and I did, so I got one last year, but I've only used it twice. Once was because of pain in the backs of my knees. Lately—not that you asked—they feel as though a big burly guy whacked them with a metal stick. But I am not an A-list ice skater aiming for the Olympics, so I guess it's just the peripheral neuropathy, or perhaps arthritis; many have the double whammy: peripheral neuropathy and arthritis. Double your trouble, not double your fun.

I know it's impossible for people with serious varieties of neuropathy to control their physical symptoms, but they can control their minds. Lt. Col. Eugene Richardson, USA Retired, one of the most knowledgeable group leaders in the country, would say, "Don't worry about the pain you might be in tomorrow. You might miss today." He is right.

—*Mims Cushing*

Acknowledgments

Follow your inner heart and the world moves in and helps.
—JOSEPH CAMPBELL

People came on board in droves to join me in this book-making adventure. They made it joyful, despite the sometimes heart-wrenching stories I received.

My thanks go to Norman Latov, MD, whom I have known for almost 10 years. He supported my first book, and then (with permission) used my personal peripheral neuropathy saga in his book, *Peripheral Neuropathy: When the Numbness, Weakness, and Pain Won't Stop* (2007). *Cope* began because Demos Health, who published his book, saw my story. They asked him if maybe I'd consider writing a book on coping. He called me, and the next day the book was underway. It's pretty unusual when your doctor becomes your "book agent," so to speak.

Working with Noreen Henson, at Demos Health, has made this project a pleasure. During our first phone meeting, she said, "The neuropathy community is an underserved one," and I knew she understood. She realized millions of people are afflicted with peripheral neuropathy, and that a coping book was long overdue. Since that call, I have been so immersed in it that one day I absentmindedly put a spray can of WD-40 in the refrigerator. I'm in good company: in *Away from Her*, Julie Christie placed a frying pan in the freezer.

Special gratitude to my fellow roundtable scribes, the River City Writers: Olivia Bissell, Carolyn Evans, Jean Johnson, June Lands, and Doris Manukian. I thank them for their patience in polishing *Cope*. My typed pages often inexplicably appeared on my desk riddled with grammar crimes, due to mysterious elves who messed up my writing while I slept after writing for 14 hours straight.

Tremendous thanks to Lt. Col. Eugene Richardson, USA Retired, M.Div., M.S., E.D.M., an inspired neuropathy support group leader, for having read an early draft and for painstakingly clarifying many points. In strengthening the book, he set me straight on the more serious types of neuropathy. He is a gifted teacher and communicator, and I appreciate his work and sense of humor. He has written hundreds of pages on the topic of neuropathy directed to the VA, the government, the media, and to his support group members.

I am forever in awe of the tireless work that neuropathy support group leaders such as Richardson do in the name of finding treatment options and aids for people with peripheral neuropathy. Bob Williamson, from Virginia Beach, is another support group leader whose newsletters are fountains of information. Enormous thanks to California's impressive Neuropathy Association support group leaders Bev Anderson from Colfax and Martha Chandley from West Sacramento. They do so much more than lead groups. Our computers talked to each other often, and they sustained me throughout the writing process. And thanks also to Sam Grundfest, who sends out energetic newsletters from Lake Worth, Florida.

Bouquets to my friend Irene Beer, a dedicated Neuropathy Association volunteer, for putting out the call that *Cope* was being hatched. She invited group leaders to contribute their personal stories and tips and to pass the word to their members. When Irene Beer talks, people listen.

Thanks also to my friend and computer expert, Lucille Devlin, who could tell by my voice that I was having a meltdown over a computer malfunction. I couldn't have done this without her technical assistance. I am also grateful to Vaughan Walker, Robert Schnitzer, Carole Salinas, and Carolyn Evans for reading *Cope* at different stages and offering their expertise. My son, Jay Keeshan, kept me supplied with hard copies when my printer developed asthma and, to my amazement, he proofread the final draft during his beloved boating season.

My thanks for sharing in the book excitement go to my daughter, my sunshine, sweet Melissa Coughlin who, along with Jay, has filled my gratitude journals for almost 40 years. And love also to son-in-law Dave, World's-Best-Daddy. You and Mel have given me my three cherished granddaughters, Schuyler, Kallianne, and Mackenzie, whose giggles make my heart overflow. If I could have chosen my children and grands, I would have chosen you all.

I am so grateful that my sister, my soul mate, Sibby DeForest, recommended that I ask people to "write their stories." That suggestion has made all the difference.

Finally, deepest regards go to those PNers who shared their stories. They have written with honesty and courage about their frustrations, pain, challenges, and, finally, their peace with it. I am honored to have met them, albeit mostly via e-mail. We have a bond that will endure. Here is a list of them in alphabetical order:

Go Team Neuropathy!

Beverly Anderson, Colfax, California
Irene H. Beer, New York City, New York
Martha Chandley, West Sacramento, California
Howard Ettlinger, Jacksonville, Florida
Ron Gedney, Jacksonville, Florida
Shane Gibbs, Wagga Wagga, Australia
Lorraine McLaughlin, Orange Park, Florida
Clifford Meyer, Citrus Valley, California
Terry Rees, Yreka, California
Eugene Richardson, Lake Placid, Florida
Fred Roberts, Jacksonville, Florida
Teri Tura, Gibraltar
Denise Weaver, Jacksonville, Florida
Robert M. Williamson, Virginia Beach, Virginia

Any sorrow can be borne if you can turn it into a story.
—Isak Dinesen

Introduction

Peripheral Neuropathy: The Most Common Disease You've Never Heard Of.
—Seen on tee shirts sold at Neuropathy Association get-togethers

What This Book Is About and Why You Should Read It

Over the course of a decade, because of the Jacksonville Peripheral Neuropathy Support Group, which I started in 1999 and headed until 2004, I've come to know people with the simple garden-variety kinds of peripheral neuropathy and the severely disabling types as well. People with neuropathy suffering from strange symptoms and who are sometimes in severe pain often have the best attitude. They cheer up anybody with or without neuropathy. This fascinates me. It is, among other things, what motivated me to write this book.

Because of *Cope*, I am linked via e-mail to dozens of people from all over the world who have neuropathy. We are connected by common neuropathy dilemmas: insufficient awareness, demeaning attitudes by "outsiders," and too little useful advice. Although The Neuropathy Association has made enormous strides from a publicity and outreach standpoint, there are still miles to go. I am hopeful this book will help you on three different levels:

Level One: That the medical information from Dr. Latov will explain how physicians approach the diagnosis and treatment of neuropathy, and answer some frequently asked questions that people have. These are meant to complement the medical information provided in his book *Peripheral Neuropathy: When the Numbness, Weakness, and Pain Won't Stop*, part of the American Academy of Neurology Press Quality of Life Guide Series.

Level Two: That the tips, which number more than 365—one for every day of the year—will help you. They have been gathered from many sources. The tips burst into my home by the dozens via e-mail. Suggestions came from exercise trainers, professionals specializing in many different fields, lecturers, neurologists, caretakers, books, and other resources. You'll find tips for wellness that have taken people—including me—years to figure out.

Level Three: That the personal histories written by people with peripheral neuropathy will inspire and further educate you about this confusing disease. The men and women in this chapter have agreed to have a by-line attached to their stories. In other instances, with the exception of support group leaders, I have changed names or eliminated last names to protect peoples' privacy.

Incidentally, I use the phrase "PNers," which was coined by author John Senneff. It makes you feel you're part of a club: the fraternal order of PNers. Someone once wrote about me, "She suffers from neuropathy." I hated that. I don't want peripheral neuropathy gremlins to have the satisfaction of thinking I'm suffering. When my feet misbehave, I call them "Bad Dogs." Me, I am simply a PNer. There are, however, many people who are in serious pain from neuropathy, who really are sufferers.

Perhaps you've been newly diagnosed with peripheral neuropathy, or maybe you haven't. Did you read an article about "burning, tingling, stabbing, pains in the feet"? It's important that you know that many more sites in your body, anywhere peripheral nerves are located, can become involved.

Bev Anderson, president of the Northern California Chapter of The Neuropathy Association, e-mailed me, "I hope the book won't be concentrated on diabetics, because they are not representative of the whole neuropathy community. One time, almost 400 people showed up for a support group meeting. It was standing room only. At that session, approximately 12 people in the audience had diabetes."

Yes, Bev, the book focuses on everyone. If people have heard of neuropathy, they often associate it with diabetes. Sixteen million people have diabetes and of those, 8 million have neuropathic pain. Of all the people with neuropathy in this country, approximately 43% have diabetic neuropathy; the other two-thirds have neuropathy because of inflammatory, nutritional, hereditary, or other reasons (see Frequently Asked Questions). Furthermore, more than 100 types of peripheral neuropathy exist.

While *Cope* is primarily for the person who struggles for answers and prays for a cure, it's for others too: it's for the spouse, the friend, the relative, and the co-worker, all of whom are baffled by neuropathy—who just don't get it. They don't get it that a person can seem to walk more or less normally, yet their feet are on fire. They don't get it that a person with neuropathy can play tennis or go for a long walk one day, yet be flattened the next. The only people who really understand it, who "get it," are those with neuropathy. So, when you're finished reading this, hand it to someone in your life who has been less than understanding. Give it to him or her at a teachable moment. Neuropathy is so misunderstood. That needs to end.

As the majority of people are diagnosed with the "numb toes, tingling, and pain" type of peripheral neuropathy, the book's focus is largely on the feet and aimed at those whose neuropathy is smoldering. No need to call 911. Firemen aren't needed to put out the flames. This is, however, also written for people with all kinds of neuropathic problems that are aflame continuously.

It is written for people who aren't sure of what they'll be able to do or not do on any given day. I salute those who suffer, and who can't do everything they once did, and I also cheer on those whose neuropathy is minimal, but who are looking for ways to improve their quality of life. Whatever reasons have drawn you to this book, I hope reading it will be of value. If we can provide a shortcut to your wellness, the book will be worthwhile for you.

If you want to add to these tips please write to: Mims Cushing, P.O. Box 3416, Ponte Vedra Beach, FL 32004–3416. I will be happy to acknowledge and give you credit for your stories or comments in a future edition of this book. If you would like a response, please include your e-mail address. You can visit my website at www.youcancopewithneuropathy.com. Your comments are welcomed.

1

Peripheral Neuropathy: Getting the Scoop

Mims Cushing

That which does not kill us makes us stronger.
—FRIEDRICH NIETZSCHE

On the Road to Understanding Peripheral Neuropathy

It's 6:00 P.M. and the front door slams. Your daughter, granddaughter, friend, or sister flops down in a chair and groans. "Oh, God, my feet are killing me!" She flings off her high heels, and you take a good look at her shoes. You would kill for them. They aren't $850 Pradas or Manolo Blahniks. She probably paid $30 for them at a discount store. They're black and white with a matching bow and 3-, maybe 4-inch high heels. So adorable, so fashionable, so in. And so not in your closet.

She sits, rubbing her feet, wiggling them, and talks about her day. In 10 minutes, she walks into the kitchen for a burrito, and that's the end of what she likes to call her "monster pain."

Whether you are male or female, you may have noticed for the past few weeks that your feet are burning. Welcome to the world of strange symptoms. Your feet may feel sunburned, but it's only February and you haven't been out in the sun. You feel stinging or electrical shocks in your toes and on the soles of your feet or even in other parts of your body. The pain escalates at night when you climb into bed, or your foot bones ache when you walk. Maybe you can't move your feet properly, or your hands are difficult to control.

You used to fall asleep easily. You've tried over-the-counter pain remedies, but they don't work, and the darnedest thing is it's uncomfortable having a bedcover on your feet. *What's going on?*

1

Symptoms of Peripheral Neuropathy

If your feet or other parts of your body bother you at night—burning, stabbing, electrical pain—but not so much in the morning, it could possibly be peripheral neuropathy.

If you put on smooth, clean leather shoes and it feels as though you are walking on hundreds of grains of sand, it could be peripheral neuropathy.

Maybe you've also begun to notice a weird tingling. *What on earth is this?* And, although you may try to deny it, you're aware of bizarre shooting pains in your feet, or even in your arms, bones, skin, or back. If these pains are focused on your feet, you might think, *I must be wearing the wrong shoes.* So you go around barefoot.

You are exhausted. You have no stamina. The strange sensations don't stop. *Can this be a food allergy? If so, what do I stop eating?* People ask you, "How can your feet be numb and cause you pain, too?" I tell them to think of their feet as one of the states in the United States, say, Vermont. In that state, it can be raining, snowing, sunny, sleeting, and windy all in the same hour, or at least in the same day. The feet are the same way.

You've heard that diabetics often have foot troubles, but you're not a diabetic. You wonder, *What should I do? What is wrong with me? Am I losing my mind?* The answer, again, could be damage to the peripheral nerves. You may remember from eighth grade science that your nervous system is divided into two parts: the *central nervous system*, which consists of nerves of the brain and spinal cord; and the peripheral nerves, which encompass all other nerves in the body. These *peripheral nerves* transmit information from the brain and spinal cord to every other part of the body, including your face, torso, digestive system, organs, some muscle groups, and cranial nerves. The peripheral nervous system allows you to move your muscles via *muscle neurons*. It also transmits sensations like temperature, touch, and pain via the *sensory neurons* to your brain. Those nerves that allow you to breathe and digest are also part of the peripheral nervous system.

What causes neuropathy? It can be caused by direct damage to the nerve, for instance, if you are injured in a sports accident or car crash. Diabetes, arthritis, lupus, Lyme's disease, alcoholism, or even viral infections (such as herpes [shingles]), can be responsible. Pressure on a nerve (as occurs in carpal tunnel syndrome) or an abnormal growth can cause damage. You might have been exposed to poisons or medicines. Cancer and HIV—both as illnesses and because of the agents used to treat them—can be sources of nerve damage. A lack of vitamin B_{12} or minerals could be the problem. Still other neuropathies are inherited, and others result from a person's own immune system attacking his or her nerves. Some types of peripheral neuropathy don't involve pain, but if yours does, or if you have other symptoms or concerns, it's time to see a doctor.

As mentioned previously, in 1996, I felt like my toes and feet were having a nervous breakdown, no pun intended. Little information was available. The Neuropathy Association was in its infancy. There was no website, no newsletter, and precious little had been written about peripheral neuropathy. Even today, if you ask ten people if they know what peripheral neuropathy is, most of them will shrug. And yet, The Neuropathy Association says 20 million people in America have peripheral neuropathy. Twenty million—that's around 6% of the total U.S. population. Poor old peripheral neuropathy doesn't get much play in the news. Its mysterious symptoms baffle some doctors, although a great number of committed medical professionals are researching this and other neurological issues.

Peripheral neuropathy is not simply a foot problem, but one that can affect the whole neuromuscular system. It's not easy to diagnose or treat. And I keep hearing people say their doctors tell them, "There's nothing we can do about it." As much as I hate to admit it, and never thought I would, if you have had a second opinion, if you have done due diligence regarding research, and if you are truly confident in your doctors, then "Go home and live your life" may be the only thing to do. That said, plenty more can be done to help you live that life, which you'll read about all through this book.

People with other ailments are told to, as Oprah might put it, "Go live your best life." The first thing you should know is this: It is extremely unlikely that you are going to die *from* it. You will die *with* it because, to date, there is no magic pill. And you may have remissions, in which the pain goes away for a while.

Peripheral Neuropathy Defined

Put in the simplest possible terms, peripheral neuropathy is damage to the peripheral nerves.

In his book, *Peripheral Neuropathy, When the Numbness, Weakness, and Pain Won't Stop*, Dr. Latov says, "Nerves have a limited capacity to heal, so it is easier to prevent or stop neuropathy from progressing than to heal it. In early or mild cases, however, neuropathy can be sometimes be reversed."[1] That tip might start you thinking about seeing a doctor sooner than you'd planned. I hope so.

Knowledge Is Important

To illustrate the prevailing lack of awareness surrounding peripheral neuropathy, I offer some information from two dictionaries. Both my user-friendly Random House *Webster's 2000 College Dictionary* and my gigantic, 2,662-page

Unabridged Webster's Third New International Dictionary do not even list peripheral neuropathy. The latter does list "peripheral neuritis" as an "inflammation of one or more peripheral nerves." Not exactly a fountain of information, is it? Now look up "neuritis": "An inflammatory or degenerative lesion of a nerve characterized by pain, sensory disturbances, paralysis, muscle atrophy, and impaired or lost reflexes in the part innervated." Eugene Richardson, Neuropathy Association support group leader and activist says, "Paralysis can be temporary or permanent, and is very common with people who suffer from the immune-mediated neuropathies, including the motor neuropathies or neuropathies due to toxins."

Neuropathy is listed in the *Unabridged Dictionary* as "Any of various abnormal states of the nervous system or nerves, especially when involving degenerative changes. Stems from a primary degeneration of nervous tissue." Dr. Latov's chapters describe neuropathy in greater detail.

If you aren't into "touchy feely" stuff, you aren't going to like hearing this, but listen up: PNers feel better if they adopt a positive attitude. In Dr. James N. Dillard's book, written with Leigh Ann Hirschman, *Chronic Pain Solution: Your Personal Path to Pain Relief: The Comprehensive, Step-by-Step Guide to Choosing the Best of Alternative and Conventional Medicine*, the authors verify this.[2] Two chapters discuss the value of distracting yourself from the pain. The best part of *Chronic Pain Solution* for PNers is, of course, the chapter on peripheral neuropathies. It's 10 pages in length.

Optimism Helps

In an article in AARP Bulletin[3] The New England Journal of Medicine was cited indicating that the single most important thing we can do for our health revolves around our personal behavior, which means that behavior, according to the *Journal*, is more important than genetics, demographics, and even health care.

People who think their life is like a glass half full, not half empty, are positive, optimistic people. They will feel better than those who are always wondering, "Why me?" and who complain. Cheerful, confident people won't be as bothered by their condition as those who are gloomy, pessimistic, or despondent due to wrong thinking and focus. Take your pick. You do have a choice as to what you think about.

What to Expect When You See Your Own Doctor

Let's say you decide your symptoms have bothered you long enough. You make an appointment with your regular internist or general practitioner (GP). (The Neuropathy Association advises all patients to schedule a visit to a neurologist for proper diagnosis and earlier detection.) You must bring in as complete a history of your symptoms as you can. Dr. Michael Pulley, neurologist with the University of Florida, says, "Some people aren't good historians. It's extremely helpful to doctors if patients are good record keepers." You don't have to make a full-time career out of journaling your pain or other symptoms, but get a log started today.

- Your log should include the following, listed across the top of the page:
  Symptoms   Date   Pain Level   Pain Relief Drugs
- That will go a long way toward helping your doctor ferret out the problem. A simple spiral-bound notebook will work fine (as opposed to loose pages or chewing gum wrappers). If you are comfortable dealing with spreadsheets, they are an excellent format for record keeping.
- Google "Pain Diary" and print out the diary developed by the American Geriatrics Society's Health in Aging at their website. It will help you record your pain, ways to alleviate it, and your level of pain. You'll impress yourself if you use it.

After a thorough check-up, your GP may suggest you see a neurologist. Depending on your level of severity, that may or may not be immediately necessary. If you can alleviate your discomfort with over-the-counter medications, fine. If you've tried them, and they've failed, perhaps you need a prescription. Don't get sucked into the "We can't do anything about it" talk until you have explored every avenue available to you. If you want more answers, seek them. And remember: Only a neurologist can accurately diagnose peripheral neuropathy.

What to Expect When You See a Neurologist

Before you choose a neurologist, talk to people in your support group and ask them to recommend a doctor. Above all, find a neurologist who is board certified in neurology and trained in neuromuscular neurology. You don't usually buy the first car you look at, so be finicky about choosing a neurologist—who will probably outlive your car. And try to find one who is a good fit with you from a personality standpoint, someone who makes you feel comfortable.

I used to think any person whose job title began with the word "neurosomething" was scary. Maybe I still do. Neurosurgeons are the docs we think about when we say, "It ain't brain surgery." These guys *do* brain surgery. A neurologist is what you need, a specialist who deals with testings and evaluations of frightening problems that other doctors may not have explanations for. And you are going to see him about tingling and burning? Yes, you are. If it's annoying, frightening, or painful enough, causing you to lose sleep, forcing you to struggle to stay employed, or changing your style of life then, yes, you are going to see a neurologist.

Bring your pain diary. Your organized history will show the doctor you're serious about your illness and she'll appreciate your coming to the point. The neurologist will want to know 10 things:

- How would you describe your symptoms?
- When did you first notice them (onset and progression)?
- Has the pain changed your quality of life? Has it worsened? Lessened? Stayed the same?
- Are you taking prescription medications? Over-the-counter ones?
- Do you take supplements?
- Do you have any other medical conditions that exist now? Ones that existed in the past?
- How are you being treated for them? What medications?
- Does anyone in your family have neuropathy, or did anyone?
- Do you have sensations in your hands that mimic those in your feet or in any other parts of your body?
- Was there an event that might be causing nerve compression?

What to Tell Your Doctor

Bob Williamson, Neuropathy Association support group leader from Virginia Beach, Virginia, reminded me about writer Dr. James Dillard's handy OPQRST system of keeping a list to show your doctor. It's another way of recording your symptoms:

O = Onset. When did the pain start?

P = Provokes. What provokes the pain?

Q = Quality. What does the pain feel like?

R = Radiates. Does the pain travel or stay in place?

S = Site. Where do you feel the pain?

T = Timing. When do you get the pain and how long does it last?

What Tests Will Be Performed?

Here's what you can expect. Your neurologist:

- Will probably do tests you've had many times in general physicals to see if your balance is intact, such as have you walk forward heel to toe. Do you wobble or can you walk straight?

- May use *quantitative sensory testing* (QST) to follow your progress and function, and use a vibrator stimulus to measure your neuropathy. He'll use a pin and lightly touch your feet in several places to see how sensitive they are, and he may use a tuning fork to test for abnormal reactions by the large nerve fibers. This vibration testing determines how quickly your feet notice the vibrations disappear. (With a normal foot, the vibrations last for a long time.)

- Will test your reflexes in the elbows and knees to see if there is a loss of motor or sensory nerves.

- Will most likely want you to have a blood test. If you have neuropathy, you may have something as simple as a vitamin B_{12} deficiency. That can be remedied and may possibly stop the neuropathy.

- May elect to schedule you for nerve conduction studies to look for large-fiber neuropathy or to perform a skin biopsy to test for small-fiber neuropathy.

Notice that I didn't say "foot pain" anywhere in this chapter's subheadings. That's because many people do not have pain and/or do not have it in their feet. It's important to emphasize that, although the majority of complaints involving neuropathy center around the feet, peripheral neuropathy—as I mentioned earlier—can affect any part of the body where peripheral nerves are located. Wherever your pain is, it's important that your doctor listens to your complaints and really hears you. When my first neurologist shook my hand to say good-bye, he said, "I'm sorry about your pain." I was disheartened. He hadn't listened. I'd never mentioned pain. I had told him, "It's not pain, it's an annoyance. It drives me nuts, and is horrible, but it's not pain." Maybe that's splitting hairs. He said there was nothing he could do, so I persisted and found help elsewhere.

Dr. Latov said, in his previous book, "If you talk to 10 people with neuropathy, you may hear 10 different sets of symptoms, but if you ask another 100, you will probably hear the same 10."

What to Ask about the Tests

Here are seven questions to ask your doctor from *Working with Your Doctor*, by Nancy Keene[4]:

- What is the purpose of the test?
- How will it contribute to diagnosis or treatment?
- What are the risks associated with this test?
- Are there simpler, less risky ways of getting this information?

- What are the side effects, and how often do they occur?
- How reliable is this test?
- How reliable is the testing facility?

Be sure to take notes and, if the doctor is talking too fast say, "Slow down!" Perhaps bring a tape recorder with you and record all this information along with the results the next time you go into the office. The best memory goes by the wayside at a doctor's office. Ask for a copy of all your medical records, especially tests. Save them.

The Doctor Says I Have Peripheral Neuropathy. Now What?

Everyone handles unpleasant medical news differently. Often, people can't even hear or process what the doctor says, which is why it's good to bring along your spouse or a friend. Some patients go into denial, while others want to know everything immediately and start surfing medical books.

For a start, do two things: go online to www.neuropathy.org, then call The Neuropathy Association at 1-888-PN-FACTS. The Neuropathy Association can refer you to a neurologist, tell you where the Association-designated neuropathy centers are, and give you the name of a support group near you. Ask to receive their ongoing neuropathy news updates. You can receive them in two ways.

The Neuropathy Association's E-Newsletter: *Neuropathy E-News*

Neuropathy E-News started in August 2007. It appears online monthly via e-mail. My feeling is that if there is something big going on with neuropathy, I'll read about it in *Neuropathy E-News* or in the *Neuropathy News* newsletter, which is surely an important reason to read them. (Sign up for *E-News* on The Neuropathy Association's home page.)

Become a Contributing Member

Send $35 to The Neuropathy Association, 60 East 42nd Street, Suite 942, New York, NY 10165, to become a contributing member, which might make your feet feel better, keep you informed, and help research get done. Or, make a donation by phone: 1-888-PN-FACTS. Mail or e-mail them the story about your neuropathy after you've had it for some time. It's a therapeutic way for you to deal with your own issues, and it helps others understand their own. Or, visit the Association's bulletin board (chat room) to connect with others and ask questions.

The Printed Neuropathy Association Newsletter: *Neuropathy News*

If you are not a fan of the web, you may prefer a printed newsletter, which has more comprehensive articles and different topics than the online version, although sometimes they overlap a bit. The newsletter also has articles by neurologists from around the country. It is delivered three times a year to all The Neuropathy Association's contributing members.

Other Resources

- Pnhelp.org is based in California. This is the website of the Northern California Chapter of The Neuropathy Association, with a link to The Neuropathy Association's website. All the information on peripheral neuropathy is clearly written and important for newcomers to neuropathy—or old-timers.
- The National Peripheral Neuropathy Community (www.npnc.org) has been in existence since 2001. It's a wonderful site, filled with energetic people on the bulletin board. It has a "Dawn Patrol" for people looking for Internet chit chat, or more likely badly needed support in the wee small hours of the morning. The NPNC's motto is "While science finds the cure, friendship will ease the pain."
- There's another bulletin board at www.neuropathy.org. These boards are invaluable for people who want to feel connected to others with peripheral neuropathy. You will learn a lot and, I hope, share a lot too.
- A free copy of Neurology Now, published by the American Academy of Neurologists, can be had by accessing www.neurology-now.com. You'll receive one free copy. If you want to subscribe for a nominal fee, call the subscriptions office at 800-422-2681. You must have a neurological disorder or be a caretaker of someone with this disorder to qualify for the free issue, which covers diseases relating to the nerves.
- IGLiving, available at www.igliving.com, is free to patients receiving intravenous immunoglobulin (IVIg) treatment for autoimmune neuropathies such as chronic inflammatory demyelinating polyneuropathy (CIDP).

If Google is your Internet browser, try "Google Alerts." Type in "Neuropathy" and you will be asked, "How often do you want to be notified?" You will be notified with information on the topic of neuropathy as often as you like. You may find the alerts to be informative and enjoy hearing what other patients have to say. Google Alerts may work with other search engines.

Conduct Your Own Internet Research

If there is one piece of advice that any smart person dealing with neuropathy would give you, it is this: Get involved with your own care. Being a docile, "good" patient is not in your best interest. That's the case with many ailments today, and neuropathy is no exception. The Internet makes it easier to do research, but surf carefully. Find the date on the Internet piece you are investigating and ask yourself: *How current is this information? Who's writing this? Is the source reliable? And, very important: Is the writer trying to sell me something?*

Managing neuropathy is difficult because not all treatments or medications benefit everyone. In fact, it's often black or white. In any given support group, some will cringe at the talk of a particular drug because they've had such rotten side effects, yet others say they can't live without it. It has "saved their life." What sense does it make that some coping solutions are poisonous to some, but heaven-sent for others? Things that seem insignificant to people without peripheral neuropathy may be an issue for PNers to deal with. Something as simple as a thin top sheet on a bed can feel like heavy burlap—it can be actually painful on one's skin.

Do Your Homework to Understand Your Peripheral Neuropathy

In the mid-1990s, Esther K. experienced all the symptoms that we now know suggest peripheral neuropathy. She went to an internist who, determining she didn't have diabetes, told her to go to a podiatrist who x-rayed her feet and had no answers for her. Next, she went to an orthopedist who prescribed orthotics, which provided no help for her at all. It is not uncommon to hear this from people who visited physicians "in the old days," which means not so long ago.

Esther continued to suffer and figured this was to be her life. Then, one day in 2001, reading the American Association of Retired People (AARP)'s magazine, Esther found her symptoms laid out in front of her, in black and white. It included an explanation of peripheral neuropathy and the advice that she should see a neurologist, which she did.

Esther had no books to turn to in the 1990s. Until recently, books on peripheral neuropathy have, with few exceptions, been restricted to pedantic, expensive medical texts directed at physicians and difficult for the layperson to comprehend. Things are turning around, at the speed of those TV tortoises, the Slowskys. I am hopeful that this will change.

So much has to change. The public has many misconceptions about peripheral neuropathy. About a week ago, my friend Madelyn told me that a friend of hers, a highly educated author and lecturer, when told that I had neuropathy, said, "Oh, well then, she must have diabetes."

"No, she doesn't," said my friend.

"But she must," this highly intelligent women repeated. And they went back and forth with Madelyn, exasperated, finally saying to her author friend, "Here's Mims's phone number. You call her." I hope she *will* call me, so I can clear up the misinformation. I will tell her neuropathy is not just for diabetics. She and millions still believe the only way you can have peripheral neuropathy is to have diabetes.

Whether you have diabetes or not, I truly believe you can live a good life with your neuropathy. Eckhart Tolle, in the Oprah-touted book, *A New Earth*, says we should make friends with our pain.[5] That may be a reach for some, but for almost every one of us, neuropathy is not life-threatening, and coping is possible. Think of your peripheral neuropathy as a badly behaved child. Put it in the time-out chair.

Common Symptoms

To sum up, here are common symptoms of peripheral neuropathy, compiled from information presented on the websites www.neuropathy.org and pnhelp.org, and from Neuropathy Association support group members :

- *Numbness*. Loss of sensation, usually starting in a toe or finger, and moving up the limb. Feels similar to Novocain, except that it doesn't wear off.

- *Burning or freezing*. Can cause annoyance or extreme pain. Skin will show a normal temperature, but you might feel as though your limbs are freezing or boiling.

- *Electrical shocks*. Sharp, intense sensations. Can come on suddenly, sporadically, and for no apparent reason.

- *Tingling*. Some describe this as feeling like having continuous pins and needles.

- *Sensitivity*. Even though you can be numb or have a loss of sensation, you can have unusual sensitivity to pressure, even light pressure. Wind blowing on you as you lie on a beach can make you want to cover yourself with a towel—and the towel can also be annoying! Bed sheets are a big nuisance to some.

- *"Stocking and glove."* Your feet may feel as though you are always wearing a stocking or a shoe. You can get into bed and think you are wearing shoes, but you are not. Your hands can feel as though you are wearing tight gloves all the time.

- *Loss of balance or coordination.* If you can't feel where your feet are, in relation to the rest of your body, you will walk abnormally. Muscles can weaken, atrophy. Tripping and falls are of concern. Climbing stairs can be very difficult.

- *Autonomic symptoms.* This is less common, but peripheral neuropathy can also upset the autonomic nerves—those that control involuntary or semi-voluntary mechanisms. This can cause vertigo, blurriness, intolerance to heat, gastrointestinal tract issues, and impotence. A majority of peripheral neuropathy patients, however, complain of problems in the limbs.

You may only have a few of these symptoms; you don't need to have every one of them to have peripheral neuropathy.

Don't give up looking for information; more valuable books are listed in the For Further Reading section.[6–9] Above all, don't lose heart; keep going. A trunk load of tips is coming up. And if you come across terms or acronyms that you don't understand, look them up in the glossary at the end of the book.

For Further Reading

1. Latov, Norman. *Peripheral Neuropathy: When the Numbness, Weakness, and Pain Won't Stop A Guide for Patients and Their Families.* New York: American Academy of Neurology/Demos Medical Publishing, 2007.

2. Dillard, James N. with Leigh Ann Hirschman. *Chronic Pain Solution: Your Personal Path to Pain Relief: The Comprehensive, Step-by-Step Guide to Choosing the Best of Alternative and Conventional Medicine.* New York: Bantam Books, 2002.

3. Smith-Liebmann, Joan. "Push prevention, not pills." AARP Bulletin, May 2008.

4. Keene, Nancy. W*orking with Your Doctor: Getting the Healthcare You Deserve.* Sebastopol: O'Reilly & Associates, 1998.

5. Tolle, Eckhart. *A New Earth.* New York: Penguin (Oprah Book Club edition), 2008.

6. Cros, Didier. *Peripheral Neuropathy: A Practical Approach to Diagnosis and Management.* Philadelphia: Lippincott Williams & Wilkins, 2001.

7. Donoghue, Paul J. and Mary Siegel. *Living With Invisible Chronic Illness: Sick and Tired of Being Sick and Tired.* New York: Norton, 1992.

8. Groopman, Jerome. *How Doctors Think.* New York: Houghton Mifflin, 2007.

9. Seneff, John A. *Numb Toes and Aching Soles: Coping With Peripheral Neuropathy.* San Antonio TX: MedPress, 1999.

2

Caring for Your Hands and Feet

Mims Cushing

*It's more important for a doctor to know the patient
than to know the patient's illness.*
—HIPPOCRATES

Your feet, indeed your whole body, will be happier if you're walking around with less weight, and therefore less pressure on your joints, heart, and so on, but let me set the record straight: You could have peripheral neuropathy and be rotund, or more politely, "well nourished," or you could be rail thin. Plenty of skinny people are saddled with peripheral neuropathy. PNers are found in all segments of the weight spectrum. Neuropathy doesn't come and zap you the day after you've eaten an entire wheel of Brie or a seven-layer, double-chocolate cake. Nor does it appear if you chow on lettuce leaves and radishes like a rabbit and are a skinnymalinkydink, a name Barbara Walters was called as a kid. (No, she doesn't have peripheral neuropathy, that I know of.) People who are 6 feet tall and change are just as likely to get peripheral neuropathy as shorties.

> Some support "groupies" of any height and weight, diabetic or not diabetic, have discovered that if they ease off sugar, they feel fewer symptoms. That's surely worth trying and certainly will be better for your body.

Want a profile of a typical PNer? There is no such thing.

- Peripheral neuropathy doesn't care if your skin color is yellow, white, red, or black.

- Whether you worship God or yourself
- Whether you live in bi-coastal mansions or city gutters
- Whether you're an army general or a corporal (but it does seem to like Vietnam vets)
- Whether you're a Rhodes scholar or kindergarten dropout
- Whether you vote for donkeys or elephants
- Whether you train for marathons or station yourself by the TV
- Whether your collar is blue or white
- Whether you smoke cocaine or gobble vitamins
- Whether you slurp pomegranate juice or margaritas (but it does seem to like alcoholics)

But the meanest thing about neuropathy? It doesn't care if you are 1 year old or pushing 80. It is an egalitarian disease. Yep, equal opportunity.

The hardest thing about writing this book is that after everything I've written, I could correctly add the qualifier "that works for some people." Because whether we're talking about wearing sandals or using a particular rub-on cream . . . you name it, if you get a group together and someone proclaims that fill-in-the-blank is drop-dead fabulous, somebody will bounce up and say, "Oh I can't use/eat/wear/do that at all!" So, do your homework, look around, experiment, and with luck you may touch on something that speaks to you.

The Foot Bone's Connected to the Ankle Bone? I Can't Feel It

In *Winning with Chronic Pain: A Complete Program for Health and Well-Being*, by Debra Fulghum Bruce, Harris H. McIlwain, and Joel C. Silverfield,[1] you'll read that in a large unnamed pain clinic, fully one-quarter of the people complained of nerve pain.

> If you had lived in Greece in the first century, physicians in "pain clinics" would have had you dunk your feet in a tub brimming with electric eels to increase your circulation. Check, please. Bioelectric medicine has improved since then, but some doctors disavow it.

In this chapter, you'll find tips on how to make your nerve pain less annoying by learning the proper care of your feet and hands, including what creams to feed them. In this first section, we'll start with socks, not shoes, because socks are baffling to many.

There's Something Funny about Socks

If you ask two people with neuropathy if they recommend socks, one will say, "I can't live without them." The other will cringe and say, "Oh my goodness me! Don't go there." Socks are a metaphor for the whole ailment. One person is 100% in one camp (regarding foot massage, medication, or treatment) and somebody else is 100% in another.

> Some PNers create a barricade or frame of PVC pipe to put under their sheet at the foot of the bed, so that bedding does not rest on their feet. Yes, even a sheet can be painful. You can also buy special support hoops sold at medical supply stores.

Medications aside, for people solidly in the "socks, you-is-my-savior camp," no pill, no elixir, no herbal supplement, lotion, salve, or oil works as well as the common, garden-variety sock (although expensive ones may feel more deluxe.) Why do others say socks drive them halfway up the wall? It's an unanswerable question. Everyone has his own unique response to sock comfort/discomfort.

If some people wear a shoe without socks for even 15 minutes, the tingling is unbearable. And some must wear socks in bed, too, summer and winter. For me, it's as though putting on socks tells my feet, "Shut up. Go to sleep. Stop bugging me." During the day, open-toed shoes or sandals are more comfortable for me. If I encase my feet in shoes with laces, it feels as though they're in prison. In Florida and other places with year-round summery climates, you might want to try wearing sandals and flip-flops, although the latter should not be worn for prolonged periods of time, or on a daily basis. Doctors have told some patients in my support group that wearing flip flops every day all summer can put too much pressure on the toes, which can lead to pain.

If you like wearing socks, PNer Bette M. offers us a suggestion: "Try Thorlo," she says. She swears by Thorlo's acrylic socks, Level 3, and found them online. The Level 3s are the thickest, and you must wear a larger shoe size. With Level 1 you don't have to buy a bigger shoe size; with Level 2, you may have to go up a size. Greg Boger of Boger Shoes in Jacksonville, Florida, says cotton isn't great if you sweat a lot. He says, "If you perspire, you don't want cotton because cotton absorbs sweat, and the sock will feel wet on your skin. Acrylic is best because it wicks away perspiration."

- People with neuropathy don't usually have sweaty feet, but if they do, they should try acrylic, not cotton, socks.

- If wearing socks offers you comfort, wear them. You do not have to check with your doctor first about wearing socks.

- Give yourself time to find socks that are right for your feet and shoes. Medipeds socks claim to be "therapeutic," ideal for diabetics because they are "non-binding, with an extra wide funnel top." The seams are smooth, and the soft, cushiony soles will not irritate your feet.

- Some thinner, lightweight socks ride low on your heels. Some are made with a small amount of stretchy spandex (Lycra) to improve comfort and fit. Some are infused with aloe. Thicker socks, with "anti-microbial technology that kills odor-causing bacteria," might work nicely with running or walking shoes. Try a variety of sock types and brands. One of them may suit you perfectly.

- Vaughan W., a PNer who worked in DuPont's Textile Fibers Department and for many years was closely involved with hosiery manufacturers for both men and boys, says, "Sock brand is a fairly reliable determinant of overall quality of construction. Brand X may use the same raw materials as Brand Y, with widely different results in the product's appearance, price, and quality of construction. So, find a brand you like and you'll want to stick with it."

Sooner or Later, You Gotta Wear Shoes

If you are a woman, neuropathy may force you to move to a less stylish shoe. Finding the right shoes drives both men and women crazy, and there's no agreeing on which style is best.

Adam Sternbergh, in his article called "You Walk Wrong," wrote that the feet of 180 humans were scrutinized in comparison to 2,000-year-old foot skeletons.[2] Scientists determined that we have wrecked our feet with *all* the different types of shoes we wear, not just stilettos or patent leather dress shoes. Among today's people, Zulus get the blue ribbon for the healthiest feet, and they go barefoot frequently. Shoes have, Sternbergh writes, wrecked our gait. If you live in this world and going barefoot is simply impossible (and often dangerous if your feet lack sensitivity), you need to have an intimate relationship with your clodhoppers, be they lace-up shoes, sandals, loafers, or cowboy boots.

The feet you put into your shoes have 26 bones. Walking puts up to 1.5 times one's body weight on the foot. Easy Spirit and New Balance, two shoe companies that sell shoes available in several widths, are a good place to start. And the passwords of the day for PNers are "wide toe box," and "rocker bottom."

The U.S. Surgeon General says it is perfectly fine to spread out your walking any way you want: 10 minutes three times a day, or 20 minutes, then 10. PNers may need to rest between walks and will be glad to know they can get in their walking. However you want to split up your goal of 30 minutes a day, walk for 30 minutes at least five times a week.

Boger's Shoes in Jacksonville, Florida, has a reputation for finding proper shoes and inserts for people with neuropathy. His family has been in the shoe business for 60 years. "Shoes and inserts may or may not offer relief. A proper fit is a good place to start. You can go to a privately owned store or chain, but it must be a place where they measure your feet. If they are numb, you can't tell whether the shoe is fitting correctly." Denise W. told me at a meeting that she hadn't been fitted for shoes since she was a kid. You need a fitting as much now as you did then.

At Boger's, Bette M. found New Balance #1123, which has a rounded toe box and is roomier for aching toes. A rocker bottom is a feature many like, with good reason: it lessens pressure on the forefront of the foot. A support group member swears by Reebok's Light Weight Gym Shoes. For just bumming around, I discovered at Dick's Sporting Goods a pair of lightweight, cushiony sandals in tricolored combinations of blues and white or tans and white. When you press your fingers into the sole, it springs back. These sandals are by Adidas and cost less than $25. They are delightfully comfortable for occasional summer wear, but you need a sturdier shoe for long walks. Find the right shoe for the right activity.

- "Inserts can often offload pressure points on your feet and will reduce the chances of ulcers," says Boger.

Shoes Are Crocs: Crocs Are Shoes

Shoes can drive you nuts and make your symptoms worse. Crocs, those funny-looking, colorful shoes that kids love, might work for you. Crocs is branching out with new styles that appeal to adults, and two styles in particular might work for people with mean feet: Crocs RX, which mold to your feet, and Crocs sandals, which are especially lightweight and comfortable. For cold weather wear, you might like to try the new Crocs with cozy, soft insoles. Look for Crocs in large department stores, sporting goods stores, or chain drug stores. Or visit www.crocs.com. Thanks to Bob Williamson for telling us about Crocs.

- Shoes that people have found helpful with neuropathy are (for women) Uggs, Birkenstock sandals, and Skechers, which have a large toe box, as well as the pricey SAS and Mephisto. For men, try Ahh Keds, Nike Air Max, Rockports, and Etonic. The Dr. Scholl's Macau Walker, according to a neuropathy bulletin board message, is very lightweight and has a Velcro closure.[3]

Barefoot: Pros and Cons (Mostly Cons)

Some people with peripheral neuropathy discover that hard floors—especially tile—give them the screaming-meemies. Cool floors make their feet feel as though frostbite is imminent. How odd is that? You'd think burning feet would like cool floors. Others say they DO love naked feet on bare floors. It's another instance of the individual nature of peripheral neuropathy symptoms.

Of course, if you have diabetes, walking around in bare feet is never, never a good idea. Diabetics have probably been told dozens of times to keep shoes on to prevent injuries. This is because, through lack of sensitivity, you could step on something nasty and not know it. In October of 2000, I attended a Diabetes Health Expo, representing our Neuropathy Self-Help Group, in the hope of getting new members. I brought a lovely crystal bowl from my home filled with samples of trail mix to lure people to our table and pick up flyers on peripheral neuropathy.

When I got home I accidentally dropped the bowl, which cracked into dozens of pieces, chunks, and slivers, all over the kitchen floor. I was barefoot. The next day, I looked at the sole of my foot, saw streaks of red, and realized I had an impressive problem. Glass was embedded in my big toe, and I hadn't known it for 18 hours. It was Saturday, but luckily my podiatrist opened his office and yanked out the offending glass. Be wary of wearing bone naked feet. Get thee to a shoe store.

- They may not be the prettiest sight, but look at your feet every day, from the bottom up.

- If you redo your floors, whether bathroom, kitchen, or garage, think about slip-resistant flooring. Whether you're barefoot or not, a slippery surface is something to avoid.

- When you drop something made of glass, sweep up the bigger pieces, then use a wet paper towel to pat gently on the floor to pick up any remaining slivers.

Don't Turn Your Feet into Popsicles

Recently I got an e-mail from a Connecticut woman I'll call Madeleine. She wrote, "In a pinch, when I have forgotten to take my meds, I use ice packs

on my feet. Today I have been on my feet a lot and my feet are on fire."
I answered her quickly, "Do not put your feet in ice or use freezing water. You
can cause a lot of damage to your nerve endings."

> Soldiers in during World War I did tremendous damage to their feet
> because they were forced to stand in freezing cold water.

You might think dunking your hot tootsies into a tub of freezing cold
water would be a good idea. Wrong. Alan Berger, MD, Professor of Neurology,
University of Florida (UF), College of Medicine-Jacksonville, and director of a
Neuropathy Association-designated medical center at UF, told his support
group to never put burning, roasting-hot feet in freezing water. It might seem
as though you are doing your feet a favor, but you are not. Warm- or cool-
water soaks are fine.

These Feet Aren't Made for Shuffling

Gail G. told a recent support group that she'd been taking some bad falls. She
couldn't figure out why, then realized she simply needed to pick up her feet.
Doing that will become a habit after a while, so start thinking about how you
walk, with every step you take. Shuffling is only permitted if you're walking in
the dark to get to your bathroom and you have a puppy who might have left a
trail of chewy bones or tennis balls that could cause you to trip.

- Falling flat on your face can give you a lousy nose job. Be aware of
  your terrain. If it's cracked, or the sidewalk is uneven, exaggerate
  your walk. You don't have to prance like a runway model, but lift
  up those feet. Let me repeat: *Pick up your feet when you walk.* Tell
  yourself to do that every time you are out and about.
- Your eyes are connected to your feet. Have your vision checked
  regularly. You need to see well to walk well.
- Give away small rugs that don't have rubber backing.
- Think about your home's lighting. Is it bright enough?
- Buy nonslip shoes.
- Avoid chairs that roll. Chairs with wheels on slippery wooden or
  tile floors can be lethal. They can slide away from you, landing you
  on the floor when you try to sit. You may miss the seat and end up
  on the floor.

Creams, Lotions, and ... Snake Oils?

The nice thing about rubbing creams onto your feet is that you probably can't harm them, and most creams and lotions don't work systemically (that is, they aren't absorbed through the skin and into the circulation; it's important to never use creams, lotions, or other substances on open sores or cuts). In the attempt to find the perfect foot cream, however, you may feel as though you're harming your wallet.

- Several people mentioned Neuragen by Origin BioMed. It is advertised in *AARP* magazine for people with chronic nerve pain and diabetic neuropathy. You apply a few drops on your feet several times a day and it's supposed to work immediately. Neuragen comes from Canada, and you can order it toll-free at 888-234-7256 or go online at www.neuragaen.com for more information.

- Aspercreme, normally used for muscle aches, can be soothing.

- Bach's Original Flower Essences, made in England, combine cherry, plum, clematis, crab apple, impatiens, rock rose, and Star of Bethlehem into a nongreasy and scent-free lotion that many find soothing.

- Capzasin has been mentioned by several support group members as one brand worth trying. The No-Mess Applicator Capzasin is a good idea because you don't get the capsaicin ointment all over your hands. If you do, *wash your hands*; it's very strong. Never use an electric heating pad with it, use it sparingly, and keep it strictly away from eyes, mouth, and mucous membranes.

- Some PNers swear by Gold Bond Foot Cream. Others like Biofreeze, Icy Hot, Super Blue Stuff, Miracle Ice, or Blue Ice brands. Usually, creams that sooth other peoples' irritated or damaged skin work well on PNers' burning feet.

- One newsletter reader claimed that Vicks VapoRub helps. It contains menthol, camphor, and eucalyptus oil, and it might relieve your nerve pain. Save it for your next cold if it doesn't help your feet.

- Support group leader Samuel Grundfast, D.D.S., from Lake Worth, Florida, e-mails long lists of tips to his support group and to many others. The tips are more oriented toward overall wellness, rather than neuropathy, but he, as a PNer himself, sometimes comes up with tips on neuropathy. At night he uses L-Arginine Cream and a pair of Nikken infrared socks. He also mentions a Biotone Peppermint Massage cream that helps feet feel better, and he's heard of people using a Thermoskin "bootie." Sam G. says, "Muscles only work when they have a healthy nerve telling them what to do. No nerve = no muscle function."

- One support group member likes arnica, an herb as old as time. Laurie Steelsmith, N.D., L.Ac., the author of *Natural Choices for Women's Health*,[4] says arnica works by lowering inflammation in bruised tissues and by strengthening the immune system. It works best on bruises and joint pain, but some people with neuropathy say it works for them. (Don't use arnica oils in aromatherapy diffusers. Pure arnica is toxic.)

- Aloe might be the one cream that fits the bill. It's the top choice with many people at various support groups. Apply aloe creams and gels liberally. You smooth it on your skin when you have a sunburn, so it isn't surprising that it works for PNers whose feet feel sunburned all the time.

- Shop around and experiment with various foot soothers. Some oils are simply snake oil, but those that aren't are pure heaven.

- Check out the product line at www.homedics.com. This company sells massaging slippers, foot massagers, and handheld massagers.

- I wish I could tell you, "Here's a massage cream that makes all the difference." I can't. It's simply a matter of trial and error. And money.

A Spa-like Home Treatment

Many PNers have feet that are extremely dry and taut. For everyday discomfort, try this: Crush six aspirins and mix with 1 tablespoon of water and 1 tablespoon of lemon juice until it reaches a paste-like consistency. Then "frost" one foot with this. Wind a warm towel around the foot, then slip a plastic bag over it, towel and all. Relax for 5–10 minutes to allow the paste to soften dry skin. Gently exfoliate with a pumice stone, then moisturize. Repeat with the other foot. You could also sleep with the bags on your feet, preferably with your feet elevated. (From *50 Ways to Ease Foot Pain*, by Suzanne M. Levine, a board certified, podiatric surgeon.[5])

- Visit www.therabathpro.com. This company is all about comfort: paraffin baths, foot comfort boots, and more.

Getting Up, Getting Out of Bed

Don't just get out of bed and start walking, because the initial sensations in your feet may be bothersome. Sit on the edge of the bed for a while and wiggle your feet. Spin them around in a circle. This might result in less morning pain, a less awkward gait, and better balance as you walk.

- Teri T., of Gibraltar, writes: "Instead of despairing about how hard it is to walk first thing in the morning, I make sure my soft slippers are at hand so I don't have to limp and struggle to the bathroom."

Nightlights

If you need to use the bathroom at night, use a nightlight. It is easy to trip over something that you can't see. If your feet lack sensitivity, you'll feel a lot more secure with an inexpensive (or fancy) nightlight or pocket flashlight.

Another good reason to use one is that your cat may be stretched out in the area between your bed and bathroom. White cat, black cat, or a cat of many colors—any pet can be a hazard in your path. Worse, your precious puppy may have created a puddle in your path. Not good for wading.

- Getting up after sitting through a long meal at a restaurant may cause dizziness, or your feet may need a moment to adjust before you stroll off. People may wonder, *What's going on? Why aren't you moving?* Martha R. has neuropathy and doesn't like to call attention to it (as so many of us do not). She doesn't like her friends or grandkids to worry, so when she first stands up, she rummages through her purse for a bit. As she does this, she wiggles her toes to wake them up. Then she is ready to walk.

Pedicures Need Not Be Painful

When choosing a pedicurist, keep hunting until you find a technician who listens to you. Most likely he or she has no knowledge of neuropathy and will think you're just ticklish. But to a PNer, a rough scrubbing can be horrible, so speak up. Look for a salon with people who listen and treat your feet gently and do not use brushes ruthlessly. You may not be able to tolerate any brushing at all. On the other hand, you may find the massage feels so good you come back for a pedicure every month.

- You are paying for your pedicure! Don't hesitate to say, "That's too rough," or "No brushes please."

Walking or Hiking Staffs

Vaughan W. has had peripheral neuropathy for 20 years and makes his own walking staff out of dead apple tree limbs and other interesting woods. He says,

- "A staff requires far less hand and wrist strength to use and has much more versatility than a cane. It is especially good for going up and down stairs, because you can reach ahead with a stick for two or more steps.

- "A staff needs to have a rubber tip to get a good grip, so you don't slip. The tips, which you can get at any hardware store, need only be replaced occasionally."

If you want to buy a walking staff, the kind that isn't curved like a peppermint cane, you can order one from Campmor for less than $40 (see Sports Seats). The L.L. Bean company sells them, too. Or, if you're good working with wood, you can make your own, and many people do just that.

Quad Canes and More

A quad cane is one with four feet. People love them because they behave. You say: "Sit. Stay." And that's what they do. A regular cane often slips to the floor with a great crash. And then you have to bend over to get it, which can be a problem if you have balance or dizziness issues. The downside is that quad canes are heavy and force you to walk more slowly, even as they offer better stability than a regular cane. You have the choice in quad canes between feet with narrower or wider widths. The wider ones are more trustworthy.

- Support group leader Bob Williamson keeps his quad cane by the bed for nighttime trips to the bathroom. He likes one or two lightweight canes for walking outside, but if his balance worsens, he plans to switch to a walker with four large wheels and a handbrake for outside.

- If you live in snow-and-ice terrain, be sure to have an ice pick–like device that screws into the bottom of your cane. Ask about this accessory at medical supply stores. Canes and ice do not mix.

- Use it, don't lose it. Your cane, that is. So, tape your name and phone number to your cane or walker so that it can be returned if it walks away from you. Ladies: Check out the straight canes in a local medical supply store, and you'll see how pretty they are. Some have a cloisonné design. And they fold down small enough to fit into a large purse. The pretty ones are great for everyday, but especially nice at a formal event when you're dressed up.

Escalators: Don't Go There

If you are new to using a cane, think before using an escalator. You're probably used to holding on to both sides of the railing; with a cane, you could get flustered. Same thing is true of a walker. Use an elevator.

Stair Lifts

You will know when it's time for you to get a stair lift installed. People with certain types of peripheral neuropathy have described their legs as "feeling as though they are encased in cement." Others say their legs "just feel heavy." Carrying things up and down stairs can be a strain. With balance issues, it can be dangerous. Falling down is bad, but falling down a flight of stairs can be ruinous. At a cost of a few thousand dollars, stair lifts are pricey, but in some cases your insurance might pay for part of it. Medicare will pay much of the cost. Check under "Durable Medical Equipment," which includes oxygen, wheelchairs, etc.

- Look into a stair lift if you are prone to falling. You don't have to be a certain age to arrange for one in your home.

Sports Seats

The kindest thing you can do for your feet is to buy a sport seat if you stand a good deal. They fold up, are lightweight, and will save you agony in many ways: if you attend your kid's soccer games, if you're a museum cruiser, or if you must wait in long lines. The seat (more like a stool) opens easily and can hold up to 250 pounds. It has no arms, but three legs. Be careful if you have poor balance or if the seat isn't wide enough for you. If you get a chance to try it first, do sit on one. They are not all alike.

- Sports seats can be found on the Internet and in some sports stores. Campmor sells them starting at under $10 on up to $40. Personally, I have found the more expensive ones to be worth it as they are more stable. So, if you have champagne taste, live large and go for the deluxe sports seat. To order by phone, call 888-226-7667 or 800-525-4784, or visit www.campmor.com. Sport seats also function as a walking stick because they feature a handhold, and when you're ready to sit it's there for you.

- PNers aren't the only people who swear by sports seats. People of all ages use them when they don't want to lug around a beach chair. People in museums will envy you.

- *Be sure to sit with the handle in front of you.* You'll feel much more secure; besides, you can topple over if you sit with the handle behind you.

Restless Leg Syndrome

Restless leg syndrome (RLS) is another form of neuropathy. According to the article "Calm Restless Legs," in the March 2008 edition of Natural Solutions magazine,[6] 12 million people suffer from it. Marilyn A. says it's extremely annoying when she sits or lies down. "My legs just want to move," she says, "I don't understand it." And neither do many doctors. If people in the 1800s complained of it, they were sometimes considered deranged and sent to an institution, but because of a tidal wave of recent research, this ailment is getting a lot more attention and, finally, the respect it deserves.

In a local newsletter for people in the Tidewater area neuropathy support group, I read about a bizarre remedy that sounds folkloric: put a bar of soap (not Dial or Dove, it says) under the sheet beneath your legs. The funny thing is, half an hour after seeing that tidbit, I read in different newsletter from a PNer who claims Dial soap under the covers works wonders!

I bring this up because it's an example of the sometimes confounding anecdotal material that is out there, whether it's dealing with cancer, neuropathy, or any other medical ailment. A bar of soap isn't going to hurt you, but be cautious with other suggestions you read about. The 2006 book, *Restless Legs Syndrome: Relief and Hope for Sleepless Victims of a Hidden Epidemic*, by Robert H. Yoakum,[7] provides more substantiated advice to help you. Restless legs syndrome may have various causes, including sleep apnea, so talk to your doctor if you experience these odd, irritating symptoms. For some people, medications are available to help quiet restless legs and other painful symptoms that interrupt sleep.

Some Alternatives

According to Roizen and Oz in their book, *You: The Smart Patient*,[8] Americans spend about $50 billion annually in alternative medical treatments. A staggering figure. The good doctors say that alternative medicine includes everything from vitamins to acupuncture, herbal medicines, massages, hypnosis, and chiropractors. These are called CAM—complementary and alternative methods—and a lot of die-hard, avid CAM fans are out there. Support group leader Sam Grundfast avoids drugs in favor of self-healing through naturalistic methods. He takes 25 supplements and vitamins a day, but he's quick to say that's not for everyone.

Roizen and Oz add that three out of four patients go for alternatives rather than (or in conjunction with) conventional treatments by a physician.

Only one in five, they say, tell their doctor about the alternative treatments they are using.

- You must tell your doctor what supplements you use because a combination of prescriptions drugs plus the vitamins, herbs, or other supplements in your shopping cart could result in system-wide, big trouble in your body.

- Collaborate with your physician when you've heard through the grapevine about a treatment or supplement. Usually the word spreads anecdotally about a supplement, and people try it even though there hasn't been much or any research on it. Clinical trials cost tremendous amounts of money and time, but if it suits you to jump the gun and try something, proceed with caution, hand in hand with your doc.

- Acupuncture, acupressure, biofeedback, magnets—all these are alternatives to conventional medicine. Some people can't live without them, others dismiss them as useless. Each one has anecdotal evidence for and against it. Support group members' reports are always mixed when it comes to results for the treatment of nerve pain—whether conventional or alternative.

Here are a couple of alternatives to conventional medicine that may, could, or, possibly, might—note the qualifiers—help.

Acupuncture

The famous Dr. Andrew Weill, author of *8 Weeks to Optimum Health*, has stated that yes, acupuncture lessens peripheral neuropathy pain, and so can reflexology.[9] It's up to you to sort through these treatment modalities and zoom in on one that you've researched diligently and feels right to you. Acupressure is in vogue now too.

Anodyne Therapy Systems

In 1994, the U.S. Food and Drug Administration (FDA) cleared Anodyne Therapy to help increase circulation (temporarily) and to decrease pain (temporarily), and also to lessen stiffness and muscle spasm. What is it? The people at Anodyne explain that the therapy uses infrared light, which is administered to affected areas of the body through special therapy pads. One of the 6,000 therapy care providers in the United States will help you try out the system, which you must do before purchasing it. You should also have physical therapy concurrently with Anodyne Therapy.

The home system can be rented on a 2-month trial basis, for a few hundred dollars. It costs a bundle to buy, around $2,000, but you can finance it for a small amount each month. Now, the big question: Does it work? Ron J. from Texas says a friend bought the equipment, and it didn't help her neuropathy. Her feet are completely numb. Ron himself had 12 sessions and found it only provided short-term relief, so he gave it up. That said, here's Grant W's story: He had skied for 60 years and was diagnosed with peripheral neuropathy in 1997. He began to have a lot of "face plants," in which he'd end up face down in the snow. Then he discovered Anodyne and is able to ski successfully again. He even skis a challenging Black Diamond run.

A woman named Sandy V. is also sold on it. After being diagnosed with peripheral neuropathy and given meds, which made her, in her word, "cuckaloo," she tried it. After three treatments, she could walk without an assistive device, and her feet were once again able to feel the pedals in her car. She has driven comfortably ever since then. After seven treatments, she bought a unit and used it a few times a week, then once a week, then tapered off, using it every now and then, following a flare-up. She says, "Anodyne played a major role in improving my quality of life." As Sandy puts it, "peripheral neuropathy is a nuisance I can live with." In addition to the Anodyne, she has worked hard to control her peripheral neuropathy through dieting and exercise.

- Some people say they use the pads just before bedtime and it helps them fall asleep. Based on the responses seen on The Neuropathy Association's bulletin board, the bottom line seems to be that some have had some luck with it, and others have not. To read more about Anodyne, check out the website at www.anodyne therapy.com.

Transcutaneous Electrical Nerve Stimulation

Transcutaneous electrical nerve stimulation (TENS) uses an electric current applied to nerves in the feet and legs to block pain messages to the brain. It can be done at a physical therapist's office or at home. Some believe that it stimulates the body to produce natural painkillers (endorphins) and thus relieve discomfort. TENS is not painful, and some have said it works. TENS is also used for many other ailments, such as tendonitis.

Cold Laser Therapy

Betsy M., of Portola Valley, California, who has mild neuropathy, asked me if I'd heard of cold laser therapy. It stimulates the body's "acupoints" in the same way that needles do in acupuncture. She is taking treatments from a physical therapist in Napa. You may want to investigate this new therapy. Try Googling it on the web.

Orthotics

Orthotics are custom-made supports for the feet, ankles, and legs. The vast majority of neuropathy patients needing orthotics have drop foot; for them, orthotics provide support, relieve pressure on part of the foot, put the foot into a better position, and ameliorate symptoms. If you have problems with dorsiflexion at the ankles, or have trouble lifting your toes up as you walk, you may find an orthotic device helpful. Orthotic supports can also be used to treat flat feet or problems in pronation.

To make a custom orthotic, a podiatrist, orthopedist, or certified orthoticist casts impressions of your feet and makes the orthotic from this mold. Depending on the problem to be corrected, an orthotic can be soft or semi-rigid. They are made to order in various materials: felt pads, cork, molded nylon, plastic, closed-cell polyethylene, or closed-cell rubber, as well as cork, viscoelastic, or silicone. The devices come in various lengths and sizes and are made to fit comfortably in your shoes; optimally, you should be able to transfer a custom orthotic among many of your shoes and boots, as you wear them. Sometimes metatarsal pads or wedges for your heels are a part of the correction.

- One Web site called orthotics "eyeglasses for the feet." Just as you need to have your eyeglasses adjusted to fit your face, you may need to have your orthotics refitted. That is a good reason to avoid lower-priced, online orthotics—who will refit them for you?

- Do not give up if you have discomfort with your initial experience. Go back to your provider and insist on a refit or adjustment. You won't wear them if they give you a headache ... um ... foot ache.

- Correctly fit to foot and ankle, the orthotic device should position the foot so that it will "sit" in a better position and enable someone with drop foot to walk more normally. Getting involved with orthotics too quickly after your symptoms appear can result in weakening your muscles, so consult with your doctor before resorting to a supportive device.

- Arch supports or insoles sold over the counter are not orthotics. They might, however, provide comfort and support for your foot.

- Alan Berger, MD, recommended the website www.ordesignslv.com because, if you click on all the subtopics, you'll find a good deal of information on orthotics. Ortho Rehab Designs is located in Las Vegas, so some people actually go there to get their orthotics ... and maybe try to pay for them with blackjack winnings. The Ortho

Rehab Designs company designs dynamic (flexible) bracing for many neurological disorders and balancing issues.

Give Your Hands a Helping Hand

The hands are sometimes affected when peripheral neuropathy, which usually starts in the feet, goes up to the knees and, as Jacksonville's Dr. Michael Pulley says, "jumps into the hands." Some people experience hand and foot problems from the start. The majority of neuropathies have been labeled "stocking-and-glove" neuropathies, because your feet often feel as though they are wearing socks and your hands feel as though they are wearing gloves. Sometimes people describe it as a constant sensation that your hands are asleep. Julie L. finds she drops things because her loss of sensation confuses her and she doesn't know how hard to grip. As with the feet, you may feel numbness or sensitivity. The average book on neuropathy might devote only a couple of pages out of 300 to the hands, which gives you an idea of the ratio of difficulties people have with their feet versus their hands.

Eight Tips for Hands with Limited Sensation

These tips come from members of the Northern California Chapter of The Neuropathy Association:

- When you test water temperature, use a part of your body that has intact sensation, such as an elbow.
- If you smoke, be extremely careful if your fingers can't feel the cigarette.
- Look before you pick up objects. Be aware that they may be sharp.
- Use your vision to compensate for a lack of sensation.
- Before negotiating ramps, stairs, or other barriers, check them out first.
- Use rubber or leather gloves. Gloves for driving help increase friction.
- Use large-handled items. If your hands feel like you are wearing gloves, but it's just the neuropathy, you'll appreciate this tip.
- Watch and listen to weather reports and dress accordingly.

Carpal tunnel syndrome is a form of neuropathy that involves a compression of the nerves, which can be improved through skilled physical therapy or surgery. The pain starts at the base of the wrist, when the carpal nerve becomes entrapped in a "tunnel" of bone in the joint. Dr. James N. Dillard, MD, in *Alternative Medicine for Dummies*,[10] says that, if you wait too long to get your carpal tunnel taken care of, you may not get a good result. Peripheral nerves can also be entrapped by an artery or muscle, as well as by a joint.

- It can hurt both your hands and your feet if you lug weighty recycle bins from your garage or closet to the sidewalk. Buy an inexpensive dolly, put the filled bins on it, and roll them out to the curb. It's so much easier than carrying them.

Shaking Hands the Donald Trump Way

I've heard that "The Donald," refuses to shake hands because he doesn't want to share germs. If the thought of someone coming at you to shake hands too strongly makes you quake, and you're wondering, "*What should I do?*" here's a suggestion: Say, "I'd love to shake hands, but my hands aren't doing well today." At a noisy cocktail party, that might not work. Try this:

- When you are shaking hands, control the person's grip by putting your left hand on top of your right. That way you can use your left hand to kind of extricate your right hand from the handshake if it's too firm.

- Doris M. and Carolyn E. reminded me that you can extend your left hand, which usually provokes a gentler handshake, or else close your hand into a fist and do a playful jab at the other person, like Howie Mandel does. I think President Obama calls it the "fist bump." You could do a "high five," but that might look strange at a formal gala.

Change for the Better

Neuropathy makes carrying a heavy handbag or purse painful. Next time you rummage in your handbag, see if you're carrying around a lot of coins in your change purse. Take out all but $1 or $2 in change and put it in a jar. When the jar is full, redeem the change for paper money and treat yourself to something special. Lighten your bag in any way possible.

Pain-free Check Writing

Writing checks is never thrilling, and when your hands hurt, the displeasure increases.

- Ask your bank about a rubber signature stamp. They are not expensive and can make signing checks less painful. Rubber Stamps Unlimited, in Plymouth, Michigan, has such stamps. Call 888-451-7300 or visit their website at sales@thestampmaker.com.

- Get yourself a foam rubber device that slips onto a pen or pencil to make your writing devices easier to use. As with the feet, the hands should be cared for with tenderness.

About Babies and Neuropathy

- Be cautious if you are not used to handling babies and have just been diagnosed with neuropathy, especially if you're a new grand-parent. You may not be aware of the deterioration of your hand strength. Holding a squirmy little one may alert you too late to the realization that your muscles aren't working properly.

- Be vigilant climbing stairs. You may have climbed stairs easily holding your own infants, but if you now have neuropathy, there's apt to be trouble with feet and hands. Hold onto the banister with one hand and the child securely against your chest with the other, and go down or up with caution, one step with one foot, then let the other join it on that same step, and so on.

Jewelry and Button Helpers

- If your hands are affected by neuropathy, it's hard to put the clasp on short necklaces or bracelets and to button clothes. For help, visit the J. H. Smith Company website at www.jhsmithcompany .com. They have easy-on, easy-off clasps and buttoners, as well as dozens of other easy-to-use items.

- If you have problems with grip, visit www.denco.theshop.com. Click onto Denco Shop when you get into the site, and go to the page called "Easy Grip" to find a number of interesting, innovative solutions.

- Sign up at www.ArthritisToday.com to get a free e-mail newsletter with tips on living with arthritis. The same tips that make it easier for peo-ple with arthritis to function often can be applied to PNers, too.

Manicures

- A manicure isn't apt to be as rough on your hands as a pedicure can be on your feet, but watch carefully and don't let your hands be treated roughly.

- The Sportaid Nail Clipper Board has a suction-cup base to prevent it from slipping. To order one, visit www.sportaid.com. The nail clipper attaches to a sturdy base and has suction feet. Also available at the Sportaid site are foam utensil grippers, key turners, zipper pulls, knob turners, and scrub and sponge helpers (to reach hard-to-get-to places). All of these might help PNers who have neuropathy in their hands. Sportaid also has an assortment of wheelchairs and much more.

Hand Helper Exercise

Therapists at Ponte Vedra Physical Therapy, Inc. in Florida say that if you type for long periods of time, occasionally stretch your hands as you sit at the computer. Do this with neuropathy (or without it), after you've typed for 30 minutes or so, or after doing any kind of work involving repetitive finger movements. Stretch your arms straight out in front of you, interlock your fingers, and invert your hands so that your palms are facing away from you. Hold that for 10 seconds. Repeat five times. And, by the way, if you sit a lot, walk around every half hour for your back. This will also help the circulation in your feet.

Something to Ponder

Let's play a little game: How many people in the United States have peripheral neuropathy?

   A. 2 million

   B. 5 million

   C. 10 million

   D. 20 million

If you've been taking copious notes, you will know the answer is D, 20 million. Congratulations, you have won $500,000. Do not pass Go without putting the money into research for peripheral neuropathy, thank you very much.

Now here's question number two, for $1 million: How many people in the United State have multiple sclerosis (MS)?

   A. 1 million

   B. 2 million

   C. 35,000

   D. 400,000

The answer is, again, D, 400,000.

Now, which disease have most people heard of? No doubt, MS.

These two different neurological diseases share many, many symptoms. People who have severe MS have a devastating illness, which can be difficult to control. People with severe peripheral neuropathy have to deal with ongoing, debilitating pain, which forces them to leave their jobs and isolates them from society. On the Internet, looking for information about MS results in about 7,610,000 sites you can hit for information. Peripheral neuropathy has a goodly amount, but still paltry by comparison: 1,620,000. Just food for thought.

For Further Reading

1. Fulghum, Debra Bruce, Bruce Harris McIlwain, and Joel C. Silverfield. *Winning With Chronic Illness: A Complete Program for Health and Well-Being.* Amherst: Prometheus, 1994.

2. Sternberg, Adam. "You walk wrong." *New York Magazine*, June 23, 2008.

3. Beer, Irene. "Making life easier." *Neuropathy News®*, December 2000.

4. Steelsmith, Laurie Steelsmith. *Natural Choices for Women's Health.* New York: Three Rivers Press, 2005.

5. Levine, Suzanne M. *50 Ways to Ease Foot Pain.* Lincolnwood: Publications International, 1994.

6. Marshall, Lisa. "Calm restless legs." *Natural Solutions*, March 2008.

7. Yoakum, Robert H. *Restless Legs Syndrome: Relief and Hope for Sleepless Victims of a Hidden Epidemic.* New York: Fireside Books, Simon and Schuster, 2006.

8. Roizen, Michael, and Mehmet C. Oz, *You: The Smart Patient: The Insider's Handbook for Getting the Best Treatment.* New York: Free Press. 2006.

9. Weill, Andrew. "Today's Question: Needle Away Neuropathy." *www.drweil.com*, April 2, 2004.

10. Dillard, James and Terra Ziporyn. *Alternative Medicine for Dummies.* Foster City: IDG Books, 1998.

11. Vonhof, John. *Fixing Your Feet: Preventative Maintenance and Treatment for Foot Problem of Runners, Hikers, and Adventure Racers.* Enumclaw, WA: WinePress Publications, 1997.

3

Exercise: Working It Out

Mims Cushing

I don't participate in any sport with ambulances at the bottom of the hill.
—ERMA BOMBECK

S ome babies seem to be wearing running shoes when they emerge from their mother's womb. It's as though they've spent 9 months running laps around a track in mama's belly. They practice doing the butterfly or backstroke at night. They jump-start their life and sprint happily through life after the womb. Other babies are perfectly content wearing loafers for 9 months. They gaze around, on the lookout for a rocking chair, then settle in with a crossword puzzle in one hand and a great novel in the other. Mine was *Gone With the Wind.* Eventually the rocking chair nesters have to face the world . . . and exercise.

To boil it down to basics, you only have to take care of three little things: your body, your mind, and your soul. Piece of cake. For your mind you read, have stimulating conversations, play chess or bridge, play those brain games your kids or grandkids glue themselves to, and so on. For your soul and heart perhaps you go to church, or to a special place, literally or figuratively. If you are artistic, you create. Which leaves us with the body. Newspapers shout at us: "You are couch potatoes! You don't exercise enough!" Yoda of Star Wars put it best: "Do, or do not. There is no try."

In *Heal the Pain, Comfort the Spirit,* by Dorene O'Hara, MD,[1] she lists aerobic exercise as number one on the checklist of "To Do's for the Patient with Chronic Pain." Other valuable things she recommends:

- Keep a pain diary and/or journal.
- Give yourself a dose of laughter and a healthy dollop of sunlight.

- Practice stretching exercises, get proper rest, engage in social activities, and make time for quiet meditation. People can benefit by adding these things to their lives, particularly those who have a chronic disease.

Well-meaning people may say, "All you need is to exercise more and you'll be fine." Exercise will not cure neuropathy. The important thing is to know *how* to exercise. It may be that exercise and physical therapy (PT) can fit into the management of your illness; sometimes PT can help remove pressure on an entrapped nerve, which is the case in carpel tunnel syndrome and trigeminal neuralgia (in which facial pain is due to nerves entrapped by arteries). In other cases, entrapped nerves may require surgery to free them.

If you feel that your feet are doing you a dirty deed with every step you take, then you'll agree that walking is wonderful exercise, but that it hurts too much to try. Tell those feet, "This is unacceptable. Enough nonsense. Settle down." Don't let your feet intimidate you and run your life so that you forego exercise. Stay on your feet as much as possible. Exercise gets your blood circulating, so that more oxygen can be carried to nerve tissue, thus slowing or preventing further deterioration.

- Don't take this ailment lying down. You may find walking is like a massage for your feet and makes them feel better.
- Do not work through the pain. Stop when it hurts more than usual.

Bouncing Out of Bed

Remember, as a kid, bouncing out of bed, first thing in the morning? If you have painful, stabbing sensations or any discomfort when you wake up, sit on the edge of your bed and do gentle "get moving" stretches. Your increased circulation will bring fresh blood to your muscles. Massage your feet, and you will help both your feet and hands.

- Stretching your tendons and ligaments will aid not only your neuropathy, but also your arthritis if you have that, too. Stretches increase flexibility and elasticity.
- Think about stretching any time during the day. If your neuropathy flares up or even if it doesn't, stretching is important.

Breaking News: Breathing Is a Good Thing

As it turns out, breathing is good for you. I told my friend Susan B. how to be less bored, waiting for her poodle to "do his business" while she stands and waits on the other end of the leash. "Take deep breaths," I said. "You'll feel like you're doing something good for yourself, not just slavishly waiting for your pooch to perform." The next time she saw me she said, "Wow! That deep breathing got rid of my headaches." Simple explanation: Breathing deeply from your diaphragm promotes full oxygenation of the red blood cells. In *You Staying Young: The Owner's Manual for Extending Your Warranty*, by Roizen and Oz,[2] they write that deep breathing makes your lungs go from 97% saturation of oxygen all the way to 100%, and that 3% makes a big difference in how you feel. Breathing deeply also aids the journey of nitric oxide, a lung and blood vessel dilator, to the lungs. Your lungs and blood vessels function better when you remember to breathe deeply.

- While the song says, "Dream when you're feeling blue," try a different lyric: "Breathe when you're feeling blue."
- When you walk, take deep breaths to increase the benefits of exercise to your body.

Chair Exercises

You may be in for a shock if you join a chair exercise class thinking it's going to be a snap. Some in the class I attended were in their 70s and 80s and doing it easily, but your first try? Your body may cry out, "Do we have to do this?" Newcomers say they are surprised at how vigorous these classes are; many chair exercise regulars do warm-up exercises first. The routines are not just for those without a lot of mobility. They're for anyone. Most of the senior centers have chair exercise classes, and many PNers may benefit from the stretching these exercises provide.

Exercising in Front of the TV: No More Couch Potatoes

*In order for man to succeed in life, God provided him
with two means, education and physical activity. Not separately,
one for the soul and the other for the body, but for the two together.
With these two means, man can attain perfection.*

—PLATO

I wonder if Shigeru Miyamoto, the 55-year-old inventor of many hot Nintendo games, such as Donkey Kong and Mario, originally thought about marketing his Nintendo Wii (pronounced "we,") to people who are physically challenged. Wii, a very popular video console game, might work for people with neuropathy who have limited movement or range of motion. Although it comes with a pretty hefty in-store price tag—$250, $300, or even more if you buy it online, it is great fun for the whole family. As one print ad says, "It seals that generation gap once and for all."

It works like this: You connect it to your TV and choose a game you want to play in the Sports Package: golf, bowling, tennis, boxing, or baseball. You use a remote control, and when a ball comes toward you on the screen—let's say you've decided to play tennis—you choose the precise moment to swing the remote control with more or less the same motion you'd use if you were using a real racket. You either score or you don't. People get pretty heated over this game, and the company also provides two nifty little wrist straps, so that you and your adversary don't fling the remote control across the room by mistake. You can buy an extra remote control for additional players. (Golf and bowling you can play alone.) It's great for hand–eye coordination and is especially fun for the person who loved sports at one time, but can't play as a result of illness or injury.

Ted C. used to bowl avidly until his knee and back issues became too painful. Then, at a retirement community in Springfield, Virginia, he discovered Wii bowling and loved it. Eventually, a virtual bowling league was started, using four Wii game systems.

People at a rehab facility in Raleigh-Durham, North Carolina, have really taken to it. One man feels he has been rehabilitated mentally and physically because of the Wii game. Another person, paralyzed from the waist down, was a boxer once, but when he came to Raleigh-Durham he couldn't keep both his hands up at once because of injuries. He's so much in favor of Nintendo's boxing game on Wii that he is now optimistic that he'll be able to spar in the ring again some day. As a plus, the jabbing and punching motions are great stress relievers. Video games are no longer for kids.

Other Health Games on the Market

- Miyamoto of Nintendo has also come up with a new, interactive physical fitness game, Wii Fit, which lets you exercise by playing a virtual skiing game, tightrope walking, or soccer game—40 activities in all, including a scale/balance board. It's called "exergaming," which *USA Weekend*, June 27, 2008, called "a growing trend."[3] You need the big Nintendo console to hook up this add-on device.

- Target and other superstores sell another adjunct to Nintendo called Wii Play. It features billiards, ping-pong, fishing, a shooting range, and other sports. It comes with an extra remote to attach to the "mother ship," the Wii Nintendo System. The nice thing is you can play these Wii games in the comfort of your own home.

Being energetic makes you more energetic. The other side of the story is lethargy begets lethargy. It's hard to start an exercise program if you cleave to laziness. Say, "I am going to (swim, walk, jog) just for today at such and such a time." And then say the same thing the next day and the next and the next. (That's not easy, but surprise yourself.)

Meet Martini

Exercise physiologist Stephen Martini is a former member of President Kennedy's Council on Physical Fitness and Sports. For the past 40 years, this celebrity fitness trainer has worked with Hollywood's major motion picture stars such as Sylvester Stallone, James Caan, Lloyd Bridges, Bill Cosby, Elizabeth Taylor, and world-class athletes such as Jimmy Connors, Martina Navratilova, Sugar Ray Leonard, and a slew of others. Doctors often send their patients to him. Martini teaches a "Stretch and Strength" class at The Players Community Senior Center in Ponte Vedra Beach, Florida. He says, "Anything you do in the way of exercise is better than nothing at all. Exercise is essential for good circulation." Swimming, he says, is one of the best. What he does not recommend for people with nerve damage or other types of physical impairments is Pilates. Martini offers these tips:

- "Pilates places an awful lot of stress on the lower back, and though it's great exercise for some, it is not for everyone.

- "If people can't run, stretching and strengthening exercises would be a good alternative to use for keeping their heart strong.

- "Be careful choosing exercise videos. Be selective, and know what's right for you, based on your blood pressure, disc issues, and so on. Don't do things that involve bouncing. That could hurt your neuropathy.

- "A mix of aerobics for endurance and weight training for strength and flexibility—calisthenics, bending, stretching, twisting—would be ideal. PNers should check with a reputable physical fitness trainer to learn what to do and what not to do."

Years ago, some of our grandparents were told not to exercise if they had arthritis or other medical problems, because it would produce more wear and tear on their body. This was bad medical advice. Don't buy into that old-school thinking, much as you may want to.

Stretching

To recap, using tips collected from various Neuropathy Association support group newsletters:

- Stretching should be done slowly. Hold each stretch for 10–15 seconds, and build up to 30 seconds.

- With each stretch, exhale. Do not hold your breath.

- Do not stretch so much that it causes pain. Stretch so that you feel mild tension.

- Do stretches when you are not stressed. You should be relaxed.

- Try to perform them regularly. Work toward quality and consistency.

Silver Sneakers Fitness Program

"Just Get Up and Move." That's the motto of the nationwide Silver Sneakers program, designed by Healthways for seniors older than 65 years. The classes are "chair-based," meaning that people may use a chair if they have balance problems, so it's a good choice of activity for PNers, because participants can do the exercises while seated. The hour starts slowly, then music with just the right energy to get people moving begins and the fun starts. The teachers say even moderate exercise has been shown to reduce the risk of heart disease, diabetes, and depression. Hand weights, colorful balls, and stretch bands are all provided by Healthways, which partners with health insurance companies.[4]

- The Silver Sneakers program may be the perfect opportunity to use your time more efficiently by exercising and socializing with a group of similarly minded people. The average age of participants is 73 and, on any given day, statistics say 43,000 people across America participate in Silver Sneakers fitness classes.

- Old School P.E., out of Newport, New Hampshire, and Urban Recess, in Portland, Oregon, are programs for adults that focus on the sports we all did as kids. It's a change from a treadmill and is kind of like recess for grown-ups. Visit their web sites at www.old-schoolpe.com/mainsite or www.urbanrecess.com. As with any sports class, check out the degree of difficulty. There may be such programs in your area.

Swimming and Pool Aerobics

Florale W. of Santa Cruz, California, has been doing pool aerobics for 20 years and is convinced it's the best exercise. It offers a good amount of neuropathic pain relief from her problems: necrotizing vasculitis and polyarteritis nodosa (PAN). She says, "(I live) with the pain and numbness day in and day out. My balance needs constant work. I no longer ride my bike, and my golf game isn't the same because of balance issues." She walks 2 or 3 miles daily and takes medication for the nerve pain. Florale is one of many who find relief in the water.

You need a sport that suits you, one you like, and one that won't make your peripheral neuropathy worse. Swimming may be perfect: it's a low-impact exercise that doesn't wear out your joints and will certainly help your balance. Here are some more tips from people who have neuropathy and also from aquatics instructors:

- Use a kickboard to give your muscle groups and cardiovascular system a workout.

- Join a water-walking class. Florida aerobics instructor Kellie T. is living proof that you can streamline your body with swim aerobics and water walking.

- Water walking for 30–45 minutes is being taught by instructors at clubs and Y's everywhere. Go slowly at first, and see how your feet feel when the class is over. Pace yourself. You don't have to keep up. PNers who are prone to feeling dizzy should take water walking slowly as the turn at each end of the pool, if done too fast, can cause dizziness for a PNer.

- Start a class yourself if you have a pool and friends who want to join you. Many books list illustrated water-based exercises that you can do yourself or with others.

- Use a swim belt to exercise in deep water. Connie B. never goes into the pool without one. "And stay in the deep end," she says. "In the shallow end, when you do jumping jacks, jogging, and other moves—all of which demand constant pounding and jumping—it can be harmful to your feet."

- Be cautious using hand weights or weighted water gloves if neuropathy bothers your hands. Caution with hand weights applies to both land and sea (pool).

- Water exercise classes for people with arthritis, done in warm water at various YM/WCA pools, are good for people with neuropathy, too.

- If you really can't exercise, but love being in the water, try using "noodles," those long, rounded Styrofoam "elephant trunks" that you can sit on. They might be an enjoyable way to cool off on a hot day. Inner tubes also work well for relaxing in the water.

Aquatic Fitness Gear

Swimming Past 50, by Mel Goldstein and Dave Tanner,[5] has a section on "Dry Land Training" that advocates stretches and has numerous illustrations to teach you exactly how to do them. The authors also explain the potential of the swimmer who is older than 50, the five types of training, workout structures, and realistic goals. Correct fitness gear is an important must:

- No person with neuropathy should do pool aerobics without wearing foot gear. Hydro-fit has walking shoes, resistance gloves, mini hand buoys, flotation belts, wet vests, and aqua suits. Some people can find water-walking shoes at KMart or Wal-Mart, but Hydro-fit shoes are excellent quality. Contact them at 800-346-7295 or www.hydrofit.com.

- Even if the outdoor pool you use is heated in winter, it may not be warm enough for you. Some can't tolerate the cold air as they enter and leave the water. Neuropathy can mess with your body's thermostat. One solution is to use a warm-up water jacket that fits over your bathing suit. Sports stores carry them, as does Hydro-fit.

Tai Chi

A good choice of exercise for many PNers is tai chi (pronounced *tie-CHEE*. *Chi* means energy), which began 450 years ago in China as a method of self-defense but has since evolved into a wonderful movement exercise regimen. This is the gracefully choreographed group exercises that many of us have seen people perform in public parks. Doing the movements can help ease neuropathic problems and boost energy and mood.[6] It's done in the manner of a meditative routine with slow, dance-like movements; when you watch it being done, you feel like everyone participating is in a trance, and maybe they are. The tranquil movements are similar to those of many animals. Look for a class that is slower-paced than usual, which is a better choice for PNers. Slower, more meditative movements will increase your range of joint motion, relax your mind, and increase circulation. The movements may help your coordination, increase blood flow, and lower your stress levels.

- Tai chi will definitely help your balance, and the socializing is good for you, too.

- A cousin to tai chi is *qigong*. This ancient Chinese exercise also uses breathing in gentle movements and allows you to improve balance and build strength. Both qigong and tai chi, according to Mehmet Roizen, MD, a wellness officer at the Cleveland Clinic and noted author, help lessen your stress levels, lower your blood pressure, increase your flexibility, and improve your circulation, all of which are very important for PNers.

Treadmill? Stationary Bike?

The weather outside is not always delightful. We see downpours, watch snow extravaganzas, or face temperatures that climb to 100 degrees. Sometimes the pollen—all the yellow yuck that clings to outdoor tables and chairs—is so bad that your patio furniture develops an allergy. The solution? Indoor exercise equipment. If you love bicycling, but can't ride because of balance issues, you might enjoy using a stationary, indoor bike. Test ride one in a store. If you don't enjoy riding a bike, then a treadmill may be right for you. Treadmills are great if you want to catch up with your TiVo'd programs or reading matter.

- To read as you use your treadmill, you may want to use a large-print book or listen to Books on Tape. Robert S. says, "Listening to a good book won't help you walk faster, but it might keep you walking for a longer time, whether you're on a treadmill or walking outside."
- Go to a store that sells used sports equipment. Play It Again Sports sells new and used bikes and treadmills. You can get a reasonable deal.
- Try out a Stair Master or elliptical machine such as Body Trek, which makes you move both arms and the legs. Some people like recumbent bikes to ride while almost lying down.

Walking

Dave Barry said, "The word aerobics comes from two Greek words. 'Aero' which means 'the ability to' and 'bics' which means 'withstand great boredom.'" Sounds right to me.

On a loftier level, "Solvitur ambulando" is a Latin phrase meaning, "It is solved by walking." Walking is a great place to start with exercise, and may be the one to stay with. In a Senior Scene article by Herb Helsel in the *Florida Times-Union*, the writer cites information from Dr. Laurel Yates of Brigham and Women's Hospital, a teaching affiliate of Harvard Medical School in Boston.[7] Yates says it's never too late to latch onto a healthier lifestyle. While genetics and dumb luck are part of the reason our lives are lengthening, we need to be responsible for our wellness.

- The great philosopher and theologian, Soren Kierkegaard (1813–1855) said at the age of 34, "Above all, do not lose your desire to walk. Every day I walk myself into a state of well being and walk away from every illness. I have walked myself into the best thoughts, and I know of no thought so burdensome that one cannot walk away from it. . . . The more one sits still, the closer one comes to feeling ill. . . . Thus if one just keeps on walking, everything will be all right."

Pain or Gain?

Dr. James O'Dell, president of the American College of Rheumatology Research and Education Foundation in Atlanta, says you should switch to another exercise if you have pain right after working out. If you have pain the day after exercise, work less intensively.[8]

Walking with a Friend or an iPod

Walking can be done in a variety of ways: in silence or with an iPod, at an indoor mall or with a dog, a friend, or a group of like-minded people:

- Go to www.ava.org and find the American Volkssport Association near you if you're interested in learning about walking clubs. Call 800-830-WALK to learn about walking events. The site lists walking clubs by state and how to form a club.

- Some like to walk the same turf every day, but it's good to alternate grassy pathways with sandy ones, or go to a park or woodsy area. Don't let your walk venues become boring.

- Watch for uneven ground if your balance is faulty.

- Walking with your spouse is a great way to catch up on the day's events. Many people prefer the security of walking with someone. On the other hand, you may be happier enjoying the companionship of nature and relishing the time to think in solitude.

- No matter what sport you choose, do it at the time of day when your neuropathy is the least bothersome and when your energy level is at its highest. Many prefer to walk in the morning. Make it part of your schedule, just like brushing your teeth.

- If you walk with a buddy, it should be someone with a similar gait to yours and kindred goals.

- If you walk on your own, put your name, address, and contact number in a pocket. You could take a spill and, God forbid, need to be taken to a hospital. How would anyone identify you if you are alone and unconscious?

- Parade music is invigorating, and with a cassette player, CD player, or any brand of MP3 player, you'll step lively. Sousa marches may keep you walking for longer than you expected.

- Get a pedometer and see if you can walk 10,000 steps a day, the recommended number for fitness. Sharon T. couldn't do more than 2,000 when she started walking, but now she does 10,000 almost every day.

Keep in Mind

Some people might have said to you, "Gee, I have neuropathy, and it's no big deal. I can't imagine needing a support group for neuropathy." Good for them. They are lucky. Don't let people dismiss your peripheral neuropathy lightly or disdain it. Tell them peripheral neuropathy is real and extremely painful for some. Symptoms vary greatly from person to person, as you've already read. While some can pooh-pooh their peripheral neuropathy, on the other hand strong men and women have cried over it.

Symptoms

Some of the symptoms that people with the most severe peripheral neuropathy experience:

- Dizziness
- Numbness
- Kidney problems
- Upper body paralysis and/or limited function of the neck
- Irregular heartbeat
- Breathing difficulties
- Digestion problems with episodes of diarrhea or constipation
- Urinary problems with overflow incontinence
- A feeling that the body has turned to cement from the waist down, especially upon climbing stairs
- Sexual problems
- Erratic blood pressure
- Sensations of electric shocks and pins-and-needles over the body
- Severe loss of stamina
- Exhaustion

Peripheral neuropathy: it is what it is—for you. If your spouse or someone you love implies that neuropathy is no big deal, show them literature about it. Tell them the ailment is real, that you are doing the best you possibly can, and that you aren't asking to be coddled.

If your neuropathy is minimal and people are treating you with kid gloves, tell them to stop if you don't like that kind of solicitude. In my own case, I was being driven somewhere and the driver, my friend, said, "Can I drop you off at the front door?" I squawked and she now understands not to kid-glove me. I told her thanks, but I wanted to walk from the parking lot. I'm not a "drop-me-at-the-front-door" kind of person.

To Those Who Still Don't Understand Why the Focus on Neuropathy Is Valid

Considering that some people suffer from devastating, life-threatening illnesses, others may feel that neuropathy patients don't "deserve" the spotlight of attention on them. And yes, neuropathy is typically not a terminal illness. Some people with peripheral neuropathy are barely affected by it. But for millions, it is debilitating to the point where they must leave a job they cannot afford to quit, are using a wheelchair all the time, or must have treatments such as regular, intravenous transfusions (IVIg) every month or 6 months. Unlike many other chronic illnesses that have so much attention focused on them, and because of the long-term negative effects that the illness causes, peripheral neuropathy needs increased public awareness and many more dollars put into funds for research.

For Further Reading

1. O'Hara, Dorene. *Heal the Pain, Comfort the Spirit: The Hows and Whys of Modern Pain Treatment*. Philadelphia: University of Pennsylvania Press, 2002.

2. Roizen, Michael. F. and Mehmet C. Oz. *YOU: Staying Young: The Owner's Manual for Extending Your Warranty*. New York: Free Press, 2007.

3. Cruise, Jorge. "Try ancient qigong." *USA Weekend*, June 13–15, 2008.

4. FitzRoy, Maggie. "Program's Pitch: 'Just get up and move.'" *Shorelines, Florida Times-Union*, March 8, 2008.

5. Goldstein, Mel, and Dave Tanner. *Swimming Past 50*. Champaign, IL: Human Kinetics Publishers, 1999

6. Berthelot, Ashley. "Reaching for relief: Ancient Chinese art form used to manage neuropathy." *Neuropathy News*® newsletter, May 2007.

7. Helsel, Herb. "Walking for wellness." *Florida Times-Union*. March 6, 2008.

8. Pagan, Camille Noe. "Walking through pain." *Arthritis Today*, March/April 2008.

4

Home and Hearth: Living More Easily and Enjoyably

Mims Cushing

He is the happiest, be he king or peasant, who finds peace in his home.
—JOHANN WOLFGANG VON GOETHE

Is this the scenario at your home when you have the flu, other ailment, or a bad spell of peripheral neuropathy?

- A mound of night clothes creates moguls around your bedroom and bathroom.
- A forest of pill bottles grows on your vanity.
- Newspapers sit in sloppy piles on your chairs.
- The drinking glasses on your night table are like a glass-instruments' orchestra.
- Dishes and bowls accumulate on kitchen counters.

You may ask, "What's this chapter got to do with neuropathy?" That's easy. If you spend more time at home due to less mobility and more pain, you'll feel better if you have "thatched your cottage" before the rain falls, an old Irish saying that tells you to take care of important things before they become overwhelming. Similarly, you want to do things when your body's weather is "fair and sunny." Having a bad neuropathic spell is like having a wicked rainstorm fall into your life. You wouldn't want to work on your roof in the rain, and you aren't going to make your house shipshape when you're in pain. When you are sick, it's easier to get around and more pleasant to live in a place that is organized, neat, and clutter free.

I'm not going to go all Martha Stewart on you, but simple things can make your house safer and more comfortable. An unorganized house can add to your misery. On a day when you're starting to feel bad and you can sense pain is on the way, work around the house. Slowly spruce it up. For many, a falling barometer can be an indicator that pain is brewing. The pain from peripheral neuropathy can wax and wane, and you want to take advantage of it when it's waning. Then, when you really need to lie down or take it easy, you'll have made your surroundings pleasant.

A picked-up house will pick you up. And beyond "picking up," take a few steps to tweak it now to help you stay out of the dumps later.

- A safe house is essential. PNers need to go the extra steps to ensure that their house is safe and free of things that might cause an accident.

- Less clutter will mean fewer things to trip over, fall on, and hike through to get at what you want.

Smart Thinking

Homeowners with neuropathy who are building a new home should think about their present and future needs and, according to builders, they are.[1] PNers are requesting doorways large enough to let a wheelchair move in and out, easily accessible showers, and entrances that have no step-down. Doorknobs can be a problem for PNers with hand troubles, so they are installing lever handles instead. An anti-scald sensor to ensure that water temperature will not burn insensitive skin is important to people with sensory neuropathy. Thinking in terms of future needs for your family or for your parents is intelligent thinking. You may not be using a tub these days and may opt out of one to have a shower stall instead, but you may regret it later—a bathtub can be soothing for overused muscles. Think ahead.

Aromatherapy

- Lemon is a scent that seems to improve mood, according to researchers at the online site, www.psychoneuroendocrinology .com. Unfortunately, they did not find any value in lemon's odor regarding healing, pain, or stress. But an improvement in mood? Take it!

- *The International Journal of Neuroscience* reports that aromatherapy massage using lemon, rosemary, chamomile, and lavender helps lower anxiety and raise self-esteem in older women.[2]

Also, lavender and sandalwood oils, when sprayed into mice cages, help the nervous critters simmer down. Could work for us.

- Nice-smelling soaps are a wonderful guilty pleasure. This may strike you as froufrou, a superfluous tidbit of luxury, so ignore it. Not me. Soaps are cheaper and last longer than flowers. Soaping your hands several times a day is a must in today's germ-ridden world. Liquid pumps dispense soap in a garden of great smells: coconut, lavender, rose, honey and oatmeal, or peppermint. Every time you wash your hands with an aroma you like, it can be an emotional pick-you-up.

Bathroom Safety

- Grab bars prevent you from slipping and increase your ease getting in and out of the shower and tub. Michelle Holland works at a Medequip in Jacksonville Beach, Florida. She talked about the value of suction-cup grabbers for a tub or shower. She said, "Be careful not to use your full weight with them. They are for assist only. The kinds you affix permanently onto the tile can support you."

- Rubber mats for tub and shower are essential. Even so-called "non-slip" floor tile in a shower can be a dangerous surface.

- A no-step shower is the latest thing in home improvement. If you are redoing your bathroom, ask your designer or contractor to install a special shower with no-step and with sloped flooring for easy access. Another hot look is a sunken shower with handrails. It's stylish, functional, and easier to navigate. Also, ask for a permanent seat in the shower, so that you can sit down in a hurry if you feel dizzy or lose your balance.

- Bathtub maneuvers can be tricky, and if you feel it's so dangerous that you deny yourself a warm soak, that is a shame. If you miss the therapeutic relaxation of a bath, it is possible to install an automated device to lower you into the tub and raise you up. It comes with a high backrest and wide seat. It's fully waterproof, battery operated, and has a simple hand control along with a remote control. One such device is Archimedes Bath Lift made by First Street: For Boomers and Beyond. Contact the company at 800-289-0063 or online at www.bathliftdirect.com.

- A walk-in tub is a wonderful (although pricey) answer for people who want to take a bath. Premier Walk-In Tubs are being touted as so easy you just open the door and step in. If your legs aren't adept at climbing out of a tub, consider these walk-ins. Call the company at 800-578-2899 for more information.

- A raised, removable toilet seat is several inches taller than a regular seat. It fits over your existing one and has handles. It will be easier when you sit down. If your neuropathy goes up to your knees, it might lessen the discomfort of sitting and standing. You can also buy permanent tall seats.

If Balance Is an Issue: Five Smart Moves to Avoid Taking a Tumble

- Paint outdoor steps with paint that has grit in it.
- Use bright-colored tape on your top and bottom outdoor steps.
- Do not use slippery wax.
- Keep electric cords out of the way.
- Slow down! On trips leave early so that you don't have to rush.

Kitchen Safety

- Water on a kitchen floor can result in a fall. If you have peripheral neuropathy, your feet might not be aware of a spill near the kitchen sink. Put down an attractive non-skid throw rug to prevent falls. Rugs, however, can also cause you to slip and fall, so it is essential that you get one with a backing that grips.

- Anti-fatigue mats are cushiony blessings in the kitchen or any place where you have to stand for a long time, as they provide great relief to sore feet. Go to the nationwide store Harbor Freight, which sells them at a low price (under $10). Or visit www.antifatiguemat.com online.

- If you find that standing on your feet is painful, wasting time hunting for a utensil in an overflowing utensil drawer is downright annoying. Take things you rarely use and put them in a box in your garage marked "Graveyard for Kitchen Stuff I'll Never Use." Smarter: Take the stuff you bought at the Home and Patio Expo and haven't used in the past year to Goodwill.

- Get a few kitchen organizers at a discount or dollar store. Sort through and weed out one drawer at a time.

- Get out those old high-fat cookbooks from the '60s and earlier, and give them to Goodwill because now you are eating healthier.

- When you feel up to it, whip up casseroles, freeze them, then save them for days when cooking hurts to even think about.
- Go through your spice rack and toss anything older than a few years. Standing and staring at your spices until you find the one you need is easier if there are fewer in your collection.

Simplify, Simplify

- The best reason to get rid of clutter is that the less you have, the easier it is to clean your house. Kathryn Weber, who writes the "Around the Home" column in a local paper, says too many knick-knacks and kitsch that don't mean anything to you any more are big obstacles to proper cleaning. And don't say, "But they all mean a lot to me!" Think of the time you'll save if you don't have to clean around bric-a-brac. Weed out. Let others enjoy them.

Edit your house. Peter Walsh's book, *It's All Too Much: An Easy Plan For Living a Richer Life with Less Stuff*, will help you do that.[3] A few of his tips:

- One day a week for two weeks, take two big trash bags (not wimpy grocery bags) and fill them up. Take one to Goodwill and send the other to the garbage. Peter Walsh's overall theme is: People, you have too much excess baggage that makes your home harder to clean and weighs you down psychologically. Try to get everyone in your household to declutter.
- Walsh also says for every category of your possessions—books, videos, clothing, shoes—get rid of one item. He calls it "downsizing." You'll probably never miss the discarded items.
- If you have things belonging to other people or relatives, return them. It's hard enough to clean your own clutter without having to clean theirs, too.

General Clean-up

- If clean-up overwhelms you, start small. Take one drawer and completely dump it out on a table. That's right. Turn it upside down and get to the bottom of things. As you clean it, methodically decide: Keep or Save. *Do I use this?* If not, toss it or Goodwill it. Start in the kitchen, start in your bedroom, but start. Clean out a drawer a day.
- When I cork off, I hate the thought of my kids having to pore over endless amounts of stuff I don't use or want. Do your heirs a favor:

Ask them if they want specific objects in your house. If they say "No," believe them.

- Take a long, thoughtful look at the adorable art drawings and stories your kids brought home from grade school, cement them in your mind, and return them to their creators. They'll either love reminiscing, or they won't care and will toss them. In any case, they won't be cluttering your closets any more.

- Clean with green. You don't need to add toxins to your home, and some cleaning products do just that. Nicole Duncan says it's bad enough that you inhale this stuff, but a big percentage goes into our rivers and streams.[4] You can find all-purpose kitchen cleaners that are plant- and mineral-based and biodegradable. One cleanser in my kitchen has a coconut-based cleaning agent. Another has wild-orange and cedar-spice aroma.

- Cleaners with carcinogens and glycol ethers found in commercial products need to go. Paul McRandle, deputy editor of the National Geographic *Green Guide*, says that glycol ethers, commonly found in products that eliminate grime, can be responsible for nerve damage as they are readily absorbed into the skin.[5] At the very least, use rubber gloves.

- Be careful using:
    - Bleach or phosphoric acid. Lung irritants. Found in bleach.
    - Butyl Cellosolve. Can damage your nerves. Found in glass cleaners.
    - Phosphate. Harms rivers and lakes. Found in dishwasher detergent.

- Stick with products containing no dyes, no detergent, no bleach or perfumes.

- *Cleaning Plain and Simple*, by Donna Smallin, is loaded with great tips to help you clean before you have a rainy day (i.e., a bad patch of neuropathy).[6] This book comes up with answers on how to prioritize your chores and clever strategies to get work done efficiently.

Prettying-up Your Place

If your neuropathy finds you struggling through the day, use the following tips that the Jacksonville, Florida, Neuropathy Association support group collected over the years:

- Find your favorite scent and use diffusers or scented candles in safe containers.

- Listen to tapes or CDs of songbirds, oceans, rain. Buy a CD of those wonderful old music boxes that our ancestors had to hand crank.

- Stashing books in a garage is a sure-fire way to ruin them. A book will become yellow, bug-stained, moldy, smelly, and mildewed if it's stored in a garage or hot attic for long enough, especially if you live in the South. It doesn't take long. Used book stores and libraries won't take them, but Goodwill takes almost anything. Books that are damp, or smell of mildew or cigarettes should absolutely be thrown out. Who's going to read them?

- Here's a website for you Internet lovers: The National Association of Professional Organizers (NAPO) may be able to help you. Visit napo@napo.net or call 856-380-6828. In 2006, members of NAPO served 135,546 clients. If you have trouble slashing and burning your junk, hire someone who will.

- Martha Stewart says if your bed is crisp and neat, you are less likely to let clutter pile onto bedroom tables and chests of drawers. A little bit of tidiness goes a long way, and your bed takes up most of your bedroom, so make your bed look nice in the morning. You'll be inspired to make the rest of the room pleasing and relaxing, too.

Ain't We Got Spring?

There's magic in the air in springtime, and you can do things to keep spring in your home that will make you feel better year-round with a few tricks. They are easy, take little time, and will make you feel better. You already know you should take advantage of your days of wellness to clean house so it looks nice when you feel lousy. Here are more tips for your house:

- Keep table mats on your dining room table so it looks set. It might prevent your kids from dumping schoolbooks on it or stop people from sorting mail all over it.

- Pop a plant in the center to make your dining room look festive. Eat there instead of at your usual location. The TV will still be in place when you're finished.

- Cut up a lemon or lime, place it in a dish, and cover with water. Microwave it for a few seconds.The citrus scent will make your microwave smell spring-fresh. Toss the lemon pieces in the disposal and let it grind away the grease.

- Use Q-Tips and take a minute or two to clean between the keys of your keyboard. The keys seem to collect fuzz balls, which makes you feel like you're typing on dust kitties. Use a microfiber cloth frequently to clean your office monitor or buy antistatic, special wipes that office supply stores sell and are safe to use on LCD screens (and TV screens, too).

- Instead of cleaning out the fridge by taking everything out of it, clean shelf by shelf. Do it every couple of weeks, so that it doesn't become a huge project. And swish clean your recycle bins and garbage pails using an environmentally safe cleaner.

- Washing pillows is a must every few months, and all pillows except foam ones can be put in the washing machine as long as you are careful to read labels and follow instructions. Wash bath mats and shower curtains to avoid letting mold and mildew become a problem. While you're in the shower, check the grout to see if it needs a touch-up.

Indoor Gardening

You may not be able to do heavy-duty outdoor gardening—mowing, raking up a huge avalanche of leaves, or carrying break-your-back bags of topsoil or mulch. So, go inside. Become an indoor gardener. Plants on the inside of your house make the air cleaner, and they remove toxins such as carbon monoxide, formaldehyde, and benzene. It's possible that, at a future date, some researcher will find that these toxins, or others, have been causing our neuropathy. If you love to see things grow, indoor gardens instill a relaxing aura in any home and will give you something to focus on as you meditate.

Paul and Sarah Edwards, in their book *Working From Home*, say the best plants to remove toxins are mother-in-law's tongue, pothos, spider plants, and gerbera daisies.[7] Just one plant won't help; you need eight to 15 to make a difference. People living in big cities should pay attention to this, neuropathy or not, since cities are notorious for having problem air.

Be careful about keeping plants in your bedroom if your immune system is compromised or if you are on immunosuppressive therapy. That information comes from Louise, a long-time nurse at a major Jacksonville (Florida) hospital. She says most patients may keep flowers in their hospital rooms (transplant patients, however, may not). Christmas cactus gives off oxygen at night, making them a particularly good choice for your bedroom.

- Indoor gardening, especially creating a terrarium, is an art unto itself. It is simple to get started and adds a pleasant ambiance to any home. Use a combination of gravel and potting soil, and top it off with moss, perhaps colorful reindeer moss, and encircle the terrarium with a ribbon. Voila! You can pretty much set it and forget it, although the plants will love you if you mist them. Some don't last too long. If they look wilted—but not dead—yank out the old plants after a couple of months, bring them to your garden to recover, and start again with new plants for indoors.

- Container gardening or dish gardening is fun, too. All you need is a glass, ceramic, or clay bowl in an interesting shape; add gravel on the bottom, potting soil, and a few plants, perhaps miniature evergreens (conifers) from the cypress or pine families grouped together in a flourish.

- An indoor cactus garden can be fun, especially if you grow those cacti that produce a ready-made rainbow of mini orange, red, or yellow flowers. Cacti can be found in hardware stores, some grocery stores, and in some flower shops.

- Bottle gardens are fun, but you need to be creative to figure out how to get the plants down the bottle's neck and settle them in the earth. Close the top until the condensation disappears. The end result is quite impressive and needs little attention. Other great indoor plants are staghorn ferns and succulents.

Louise Johnson, who trained at Longwood Gardens in Pennsylvania, works at a nursery on Palm Valley Road in Palm Valley, Florida. I attended her lecture, "Thrillers, Fillers, and Spillers" and was surprised at how easy container gardening is.

- For an impressive effect, take a large clay pot, put a smaller pot upside down inside it, then put a taller pot on top of that, right side up. The "Thriller," some nice pentas, for instance, goes on top. Then you fill in the rest with trailing plants (the "Spillers") and plant "Fillers" all around. "It works beautifully in apartments or homes with a sunny spot, and will please you and your guests every time you look at it," Johnson said.

- "The Japanese are all about patience and not rushing. You can't force succulents to grow. Cacti are so easy, so popular," Johnson says, "and can survive a black thumb."

- If you want simple, easy-to-grow plants to make your home pleasant when you're in the dumps, Chinese evergreens are a snap.[8] They grow in low light *and* they help clean the air. Another choice needing minimal care is sanseveria (mother-in-law's tongue), which is happy in any light. These are sturdy, industrial-strength plants. Water them every 3 weeks, drain after half an hour; feed them 20-20-20 liquid fertilizer every 3 months. Warning to cat owners: both Chinese evergreen and sanseveria are toxic to cats, so put them well out of curious kitty's climbing reach, unless you've observed her around them for a few days and see that she ignores them.

- Bonsai can be fairly fussy to nurture, but if you enjoy the idea of having these miniature plants and landscapes in your home, look for them at specialty garden shops. If they bring a sense of peace and tranquility into your home, they are worth the expense and effort. An easier "Asian look" alternative is bamboo good-luck plants (really a variety of *Dracaena*).

Keep This in Mind

- The time you save *not* having to clean all your unneeded stuff—in, on, and around it—is time you could use to promote healthy pursuits that will help your neuropathy, such as working on your favorite hobby, walking, swimming, or bike riding (maybe on a bike with three wheels).

- The ultimate thing to throw away is your location. You might think your neuropathy is so bad in winter that a southern relocation makes sense, but approach the move with tremendous thought. Perhaps rent for a year in a dry, sunny climate before you move to Arizona for good. Some PNers are just as bothered by intense heat. You don't want to have to move back to your former home state. Rewinding is no fun.

The bottom line is that you want to be organized so that you can function more easily and efficiently on those days when cleaning seems like a gargantuan task. You don't have to eliminate every scrap of paper on your desk. Put a system in place so that you can keep your place looking comfortable and clean. Take baby steps, a room at a time, a drawer at a time, and when you're feeling crummy, you can relax and not have to scurry around looking for your checkbook or an important receipt.

For Further Reading

1. Rho, K. H., S.H. Han, K.S. Kim, and M.S. Lee. "Effects of Aromatherapy Massage on Anxiety and Self-Esteem in Korean Elderly Women. *International Journal of Neuroscience*. vol. 116, pp. 1447–1451, 2006.

2. Whittington, R.P. Designs for the times: Universal design popular with boomers. Real Estate section. *Florida Times-Union*, June 29, 2008.

3. Walsh, Peter. *It's All Too Much: An Easy Plan for Living a Richer Life with Less Stuff*. New York: Free Press, a division of Simon & Schuster, 2006

4. Duncan, Nicole. "Green, clean fun." *Natural Solutions*, April 2008.

5. Karaim, Reed. "Hazards of Home." *AARP Bulletin,* May 2008.

6. Smallin, Donna. *Cleaning Plain and Simple.* New York: Storey Books, 2006.

7. Edwards, Paul and Sarah. *Working From Home: Everything You Need to Know About Living and Working Under the Same Roof.* New York: Jeffrey Tarcher/Putnam, 1999.

8. "Foolproof Chinese evergreen." Container Gardening Issue. *Southern Living.* May 2008.

5

Wellness: Spotlighting the Positive

Mims Cushing

I am content with weaknesses, insults, hardships, persecutions, and difficulties for Christ's sake. For when I am weak, then I am strong.
—New Testament, Corinthians 2:12:10

This country has gone wild over wellness. Wellness cheerleaders say, "Don't follow the drug route. Follow the green fork in the road." A huge Wellness Center is being built for a life-care community, Fleet Landing, in the little coastal town of Atlantic Beach, Florida. Pass the pomegranate juice and sign me up. The Center will focus on six areas covered in *Cope:* vocational (I've dealt with vocational), social, intellectual, spiritual, physical, and emotional wellness.

Attitude and Other Thoughts

Attitude, with a capital A, is everything. It's not what life throws at you that matters; it's how you handle it. We have an option: Every one of us will have to deal with some kind of pain or illness. That's a given. But we can decide whether or not to bellyache about it. Bellyaching is optional.

A positive attitude is essential to Patrick Craig C., 48, of Knoxville, Tennessee. He has chronic inflammatory demyelinating polyneuropathy (CIDP), which damages the myelin sheaths of the peripheral nerves. It was eventually diagnosed through nerve biopsy in 2005, the original diagnosis having been Guillain-Barré syndrome (GBS). He has had plasma exchange and is having ongoing treatments of intravenous immunoglobulin (IVIg). Initially, the treatments left him so weak he could barely walk or stand. He is getting the same drug now, but not as frequently, and he is in remission. He still gets tremors and doesn't have his former strength or stamina. He has had to stop working and is on disability. Here are some of his tips; I like to call this Patrick Craig's List:

- Having good doctors who listen to you is essential. Ask questions and make sure they know how you feel.
- A good attitude is all important when you are at your lowest.
- Keep up with all your medical records, so that you have proof of your illness if you are trying to get disability.
- Don't ever give up, and if you need help don't be ashamed to ask. My wife, my mom, and my sister have had to bathe and dress me because I couldn't do it myself. If you need the help of a walker or a cane, use it.
- Go on line and Google other peoples' forums, other doctors, and medications to know about side effects.

Benign Neglect

In *The Extraordinary Healing Power of Ordinary Things: Fourteen Natural Steps to Health and Happiness*, by Larry Dossey, MD,[1] he talks about benign neglect and how people have often found themselves in remission because of stopping medication. You must taper off, and it must be done properly, with a doctor's advice, but there's no sense in taking meds if you don't need them. And maybe you don't.

Dr. Dossey's book is full of things we know to be true: music can make us feel better; optimism is essential; living, breathing plants should play a part in our lives; and so much more. This is a good book for your nightstand.

Brain Massage

My friend Red F. asked why brain games should be included in here. One reason is that many people with neuropathy have bouts of depression, and brain activities might get them out of a funk. The other reason is that the majority of PNers are not as physically able to participate in sports as they once did, so brain games are a sensible alternative. Blind people let their ears do the work of their eyes, and so, too, the brain can help you with the dilemmas your feet are facing.

- Ronnie L. Simmons, PhD,[2] says exercising the mind by reading books has a triple benefit: it works the brain, gives you relaxation time, and lets you relieve stress.

The brain is the hot organ du jour. It has 100 billion neurons and weighs about 3 pounds, the weight of some Yorkshire Terriers. A market researcher for Smart Brains, Alvaro Fernandez, says the brain game industry will hit $2 billion in 2015. In 2007, it was a mere $225 million.[3] Retail outlets are popping up that sell only brain fitness software, books, and board games.

Posit Science designs items strictly for the older generation. Keeping your memory sharp through mental exercise has been a big topic for years. Whether you look at freebie pamphlets or read scholarly books, you have learned about ways to spark your brain using handheld games or clicking onto the Internet's various free sites such as Great Fun Games to play board games online, solve crossword puzzles, or play bridge, Scrabble, or chess. You can work at Sudoku, take a course, or hunker down over a Rubik's cube. All are mind stimulators and distractions from your peripheral neuropathy.

- Both Yahoo.com and MSN.com have board games you can play online. I'm told MSN is better for card games.

Going back to Nintendo (discussed in Chapter 3), the Nintendo handheld gaming system is surprisingly effective because it forces players to use both sides of the brain, and doing that is doubly valuable, says Dr. Maurice Ramirez, medical officer with the U.S. Department of Homeland Security.[4] You sharpen your memory and span of attention, while taking your mind away from where your pain has settled. A global Internet information provider, comScore, Inc., discovered that 28% of players during February 2007 were 50 or older. The suggestions below can help you get your mojo going.

- Try "free samples" of brain games for an hour or a week on the Internet. After the trial, some games cost money. Proceed with caution, as a security notice might pop up on screen, telling you the site might not be secure.

- An easy-to-navigate game site can be found at www.aarp.com. You can play dozens of games such as backgammon, chess, checkers, sudoku, hangman, solitaire, and something called mahjongg toy chest. It will keep you busy for hours. (Hangman, of all things, drove me nuts!) Video games are getting smarter, and you will be, too.

- Try www.lumosity.com, where you can get a free 7-day trial. The various games you can choose keep your mind active by testing your memory and attention to visual objects that pop onto the screen. This is one concentration game that'll keep your mind off your symptoms. It's a positive addiction.

- Another game I found addictive is at www.freerice.com/index.php. It's called Free Rice, and it's the best online word game I know of.

FreeRice has a database with a gazillion words ranging from easy to challenging. When you get into the site, one word pops up. Guess the correct definition from four choices, and you may continue to play. The best thing: The more you answer correctly, the more money the site's sponsors donate to feed the poor around the world.

- A site based on a similar principle and invented by a 12-year-old girl is called www.freekibble.com. Every day that you play a game, kibble is given to starving dogs, abandoned because of house foreclosures.

Word game books abound, such as *Word-a-Holic Quiz Book: Guess the Meaning of Real Words You Won't Believe*, by Carolyn Davidson.[5] She says we use approximately the same 400 words over and over. Davidson has chosen some lulus out of the 400,000 words that suffer from cobwebs in our dictionaries. You can give your brain a workout if you memorize some of the words she has offered, such as *floccinaucinihilipilification*.

It means worthless trivia. Here's one: If you have a teenage son, you can point at him and tell him, "You are ponophobic!" He may dial 911 and say you are verbally abusing him, but you're only telling him he has a fear of work. Rather than kill some more trees on this topic, I'll let you explore quiz books on your own.

- Keep your brain healthy, because one-tenth of the cells are history by the time you reach 65. We lose 40,000 nerve cells a day, but not the peripheral ones, according to doctors Michael F. Roizen and Mehmet C. Oz in their book *You: Staying Young*.[6]
- One of billionaire Warren Buffet's passions is bridge. He calls playing bridge "mental dancing." He said in an interview on the television show, *Sunday Morning*, July 27, 2008, "If I'm playing bridge and a naked woman walks by, I won't notice."[7] Card games in general are a great way to let your brain dance. Bill Gates once said, "Bridge is so complex that computers haven't completely mastered it."[7]

Chronic Conditions: Musings

It would be nice if neuropathy gave you a warning, some advance notice. I never heard anybody say, "I think I'm coming down with neuropathy." My friend Ann La C., who is in her 70s and looks like a pixie, has never had any serious illnesses at all. How fortunate is she.

For most people, chronic conditions appear as they age. The Centers for Disease Control (CDC) says more than 80% of Americans have one chronic problem and 50% have two. Some chronic illnesses, *some* neuropathies included, can be shuffled into the background, but other forms charge full-steam ahead. You can't run away from peripheral neuropathy, fighting it just messes with your stress level, and that leaves us with one option: Go with it.

In *Love, Medicine, and Miracles*, Bernie Siegel, MD,[8] describes 20% of chronically ill people as "survivors." They initiate their own recovery by taking control of their illness and pointing themselves in a different direction. He says 60% simply let their doctors make the decisions. The remaining 20%, according to Siegel, are content to die because their lives are in shambles.

Many people don't like change. It's easier to just tell a doctor, "Fix it." You have to choose whether or not you want to be in the "survivor" category. If you are, work hand-in-hand with a doctor in whom you feel confident. As Norman Cousins wrote in *Anatomy of an Illness as Perceived by the Patient*,[9] what we want most from our doctors is time, so that they can listen and hear us, explain things that sound baffling, reassure us, and guide us to specialists whose very presence in our lives often stands for something "new and threatening."

Chronic Pain: Observations

No one can escape pain and illness. In Arthur Rosenfeld's *The Truth About Chronic Pain,* he interviews 36 people.[10] One of the most interesting is Madeline Koi Bastis, R.N. She is a Zen Buddhist priest and founder/director of the Peaceful Dwelling Project. She tells us what many PNers have discovered to be true: If you are suffering from a pain other than your neuropathy, the mind can't focus on both pains. She had an abscessed tooth and suddenly pulled a muscle in her groin. "That pain was so excruciating that my tooth didn't hurt anymore," she said. "What I found was that the mind can only handle one thing at a time."

She continues:

- "Pain is like sound. It rises and it subsides. We can't control that. What we can control is how we respond to the pain. When I get hurt, I expect the pain to ebb and flow. It's not a solid knot. If one is willing, one can really look at the quality of the pain and see it change."

- Bastis says, "I've learned there is a way of befriending the pain, of giving the pain space to exist. It is possible to live with pain and accept it."

- Look for alternatives that make you feel better: First, breathe deeply and think about what you want to do: have a massage, have a latte grande at a coffee shop and sit near the window and people-watch. Work through the books on your nightstand and choose a humdinger.

- Discover your own pocket of comfort and serenity. Lucy L. goes outside as much as possible when she's having a flare. She says, "I'm happier if I let nature in."

Complementary and Alternative Medicine

A support group leader sent me information which stated that 55% of adults said they would probably seek help from both complementary medicine, which goes along with conventional medical treatments, and alternative medicine (collectively known as CAM), such as massage, Ayurveda (which uses herbal remedies), self-hypnosis, deep relaxation, and guided visualization, which can be used in place of conventional medicine or along with it. Other alternative methods such as meditation and Reiki are listed separately.

- In a study reported in the *New York Times*[11] four methods of meditation were studied to see what the effects are on emotional and physical health:
  - Tai chi. Studies are mixed. Sometimes helps lower blood pressure; can help improve balance.
  - Transcendental meditation. Can reduce blood pressure in some patients.
  - Yoga. Studies showed mixed results, but it can lower stress.
  - Mindful meditation. This newer form of meditation can help manage pain and lessen symptoms of depression. With mindful meditation, you find a comfortable place, position yourself so you are comfortable, and focus on your breathing. It is focused awareness on what is going on around you minute by minute. You catch the painful feelings, accept them, and let them be. The writer calls it "catch and release"—you see your emotions and let them go. It is based on the teachings of Siddhartha, the fifth-century B.C. Indian prince known later as Buddha.
- Visit the National Institutes of Health's website for the National Center for Complementary and Alternative Medicine at http://nccam.nih.gov.

Depression

People are like stained glass windows: They sparkle and shine when the sun is out, but when the darkness sets in, their true beauty is revealed only if there is a light within.
—ELIZABETH KUBLER-ROSS

When you are initially diagnosed with peripheral neuropathy, you may or may not feel depressed. People normally do grieve when they are diagnosed with neuropathy, particularly if it robs them of a sport they love. If a person is suddenly unable to play tennis or ski on weekends or during vacations, it is understandable that the loss will be felt deeply. With a badly torn knee or a broken ankle—as annoying as it may be—this is a temporary nuisance. A person with peripheral neuropathy may have to restrict or limit a particular sport indefinitely, or in severe cases forego it entirely.

Perhaps exhaustion makes us less able to keep up with our children or grandchildren. Does that make us angry? It can. Lt. Col. Eugene B. Richardson, USA Retired, who is cited in many places in this book, says: "Anger can be your worst enemy when you turn it on yourself. With neuropathy, anger can sidetrack you from the goals of wellness and coping with your illness." He says you can befriend anger. "Use it to fight your disease. Don't take it out on your family or friends."

Sometimes antidepressants are prescribed, not because you are depressed, but because these meds can help ease sensory problems. These meds may also be prescribed for a combination of reasons, physical and emotional. It's important that you understand the reason for the prescription.

- Pay attention if you have symptoms of despair, hopelessness, or sadness, or if you have lost interest in relationships. If the amount you normally sleep and eat has changed, and if this continues for a couple of months, mention it to your physician. You must understand and take ownership of your neuropathy, and depression can be one facet of it.

Meditation is one of the keys to letting yourself float and stop trying to fight or flee those feelings that can be a precursor to depression. Meditation is helpful for people who are depressed because, as John Zawacki says in Bill Moyers' book *Healing and the Mind*,[12] a person who is depressed doesn't have feelings of self-love. Slowing down, becoming aware of what you have at your very core is healing in and of itself. Learning to accept yourself has tremendous power.

Family and Friends

Let us be grateful to people who make us happy;
they are the charming gardeners who make our souls blossom.
—MARCEL PROUST

Close family members and dear friends send us the best tonic. They offer the most positive vibrations and visit our homes with good cheer. You will especially need them if you are not someone who jumps easily into support groups.

- The first people to turn to after your diagnosis are those closest to you. Depending on the severity of your neuropathy, you may want to tell them how they can be helpful. Keeping up with your social connections is all important.

- As your symptoms ebb and flow, you may need help with cooking, shopping, driving to stores, and so on. Let people be helpful. It makes them feel happy.

- You may need a respite from going outside when the weather is extremely hot or cold, as temperatures can adversely affect your symptoms.

- You'd want the satisfaction of caring for your relatives or friends if they were ill; their helping you will give them satisfaction, too.

Flu Shots? Yes or No

When you go for a flu shot and are asked to fill out the release form, do you get down to the part that asks if you have neurological issues and gulp, but get the shot anyway? Should you? Are flu shots a good idea for PNers? Here's the word from Kenneth C. Gorson, MD, Tufts University of Medicine.[13] Dr. Gorson says the answer is Yes, for a large percentage of people with peripheral neuropathy, do get the shot. (But it never hurts to ask your doctor to see what she says.) Also see Dr. Latov's comments in his FAQ section.

- No evidence exists that PNers are adversely affected by the vaccine. In fact, people with diabetic peripheral neuropathy (DPN) and other types of neuropathy can find complications arise if they do get the flu, according to the CDC.[13]

- Who should stay away from the vaccine? People with immune neuropathies, such as CIDP or GBS.

- Approximately 36,000 people die from the flu every year, and 200,000 people are hospitalized.[13]

- The only good thing about getting a nasty case of the flu is that it might make you forget about your neuropathy for a while. But it's not worth it, so roll up your sleeve.

Happiness: The Best Things in Life Are Simple Pleasures

Happiness depends ... less on exterior things than most people suppose.
—WILLIAM COWPER

So much has been written on happiness and a sense of well-being. Many conclude that happiness is not about money, a corner office with windows, or a glitzy sports car. The moon does belong to everyone. It's free. The best things in life truly are free.

Coretta Scott King said she never thought money or the finer things in life made people happy. Her happiness was in being filled spiritually. Pastor John Dolaghan told the congregants at The Chapel at Sawgrass in Ponte Vedra Beach, Florida, one Sunday that, in earlier times the seven wealthiest men who ever lived either died in prison, committed suicide, or were impoverished at the end of their life.

In Eric Weiner's *The Geography of Bliss: One Grump's Search for the Happiest Places in the World*,[14] the author tells us where happiness is—and is not. America is by far the wealthiest country in the world, yet we are ranked 23rd in terms of happiness. (Another source in a television news report showed us to be 16th. Take your pick.) In any event, it's pretty amazing, isn't it? Weiner puts it this way: We are three times wealthier today than in 1950, but we are no happier. His amusing book is worth reading. It may make you feel less grumpy, perhaps even make you smile. What a concept.

- Here's the deal: You can't sit around with bated breath waiting for joy to land in your lap. Sorry, but the bluebird of happiness is otherwise occupied, probably searching the highways for road kill. Weiner saw this sign in Miami on a yellow VW Beetle convertible: "Woe isn't you. Dare to be happy." Way to go, Florida.

- In interviews with 28,000 people between the ages of 18 and 88 who participated in a "happiness" study at Duke University, 33% of Americans in their late 80s said they are very happy. Only 24% of people age 18 to their early 20s described themselves as very happy. Baby boomers are the least happy. Aging expert Linda George of Duke says these "happiness findings" are important because people often think of the latter stage of life as not being the best part. She says now people can look forward to it.[15]

- Neuropathy is not infectious. Being around happy people IS. Let cheerful people drag you up. And, if you're not around happy people, pretend to be happy. "Fake it till you make it." Smile even when your heart isn't in it, because in time it will be.

- Darrin M. McMahon, a Florida State University history professor, wrote a book called *Happiness: A History*.[16] In it he says you can't clench your fists and will yourself to be happy. You have to relax and focus on being grateful for your relationships. To me, being grateful is the secret fountain of youth. Happiness will envelope you if you don't force it. And the more you are happy, the less you will think about your pain.

Deepak Chopra's PBS special, *The Happiness Prescription*, should not be missed. Perhaps you can see it the next time around. His philosophy is that our goal of all goals should be a spiritual one. Spiritual goals are peace, laughter, harmony, love, and happiness.

He says that we think that, if we have our health, we'll be happy. But it's the other way around. If you are happy, he says, you are going to be healthier. In the words of Abraham Lincoln, "Most folks are as happy as they make up their minds to be."

The concepts of "pay it forward"—do one nice thing a day, appreciate ordinary events—can't help but make you happy. We need to do more random acts of kindness and senseless acts of love, a phrase that revved up in the mid-90s. It will take your mind off your neuropathy.

Healing Body with Mind

The book, *The Healing Mind*, by Dr. Paul Martin,[17] will convince you, if you're not already convinced, that thoughts going through your mind can affect how your body feels. This discussion has been around since olden times. Some people are thoroughly convinced of the mind–body connection, while skeptics continue to dismiss the notion. Dr. Martin acknowledges that many, especially doctors and scientists, feel it is simpler to look toward physical problems of an illness rather than to believe that "thoughts and emotions can affect our health." Keep reading and then decide for yourself.

Hope

So far, airlines aren't charging passengers for boarding with a book, so a month ago I brought with me Jerome Groopman's *The Anatomy of Hope: How People Prevail in the Face of Illness*.[18] About two-thirds of the way through his book, Groopman flew me to an amazing place.

While Dr. Groopman was in training for the Boston Marathon, he injured himself, rupturing a lumbar disc, which caused excruciating pain. His doctors struggled with how to treat him. Pain killers did nothing; he needed a discectomy. That surgery failed, causing more pain. He had a fusion, which also failed. He couldn't walk or stand.

For 19 years he lived in intolerable pain and limited himself to fewer and fewer activities. Dr. Groopman was doing what most people with pain do: He stopped activities that caused pain. He stopped walking long distances because it caused such great discomfort. He stopped lifting his children for the same reason and stopped traveling. Inertia ruled.

One day, a Dr. Rainville entered his life and completely turned his situation around. Rainville claimed that the "god of pain" is never satisfied. He said the more you give up sports, daily tasks, and things you love, the more the god of pain demands you stop activities, until your life becomes suffocated from the limitations.

Dr. Rainville told him he must not think of pain as a "red flag," because when you do that you start sacrificing everything you love as a kind of offering to the gods: *"If I stop walking, will you please stop the pain? If I stop lifting anything heavy, will you please stop the pain?"* Groopman was stunned at Rainville's suggestions. Preposterous. But Rainville persisted and said the pain would lessen the more he stopped paying attention to his disability and stopped sacrificing what he loved doing.

Well, of course Dr. G. was stunned by Dr. R.'s telling him to "Ignore the pain," which is what all those "mean" doctors have been saying to many of us: *Go live your life.* Your body gets used to the laziness you've been fostering, so you must build up slowly to remind your ligaments and muscles how to move.

Groopman, with much skepticism, paid attention to his doctor. With lengthy and arduous rehabilitation, he built up his body, strengthened it, and, in fact, stopped his "pain circuitry." He says that, even when his nerves acted up once in a while, they sent muted messages to the brain, and the fierce pain abated. It took grit and courage, but Groopman prevailed. After 1 year, Dr. Groopman awoke every day with no pain. He and others are scratching at the surface of what he calls "the biology of hope."

The idea is to challenge yourself, if your neuropathy isn't incapacitating. Your nerves will be angry at first, and moderation is the key; however, a little work every day will result in less and less pain. You are (probably) not 17 any more, so go easy.

Keep On Keeping On, and You May Run Out of Gas

Deb H. of Las Cruces, New Mexico, is in her mid-seventies. When she was young, her mother would tell her when the going was difficult, "Just keep on keeping on." It was Deb's mantra when she and her family moved all around the globe 17 times with the Army. And now, with her husband suffering from Alzheimer's disease, she is still "keeping on." A certain amount of that philosophy is good; nevertheless, there comes a point at which you need to switch gears.

If you are having a day of pain, keeping on can be a lot easier when you don't fight it. Your body is telling you to ease up. Sometimes days drag by. They creep along. *What to do ... What to do ...?* You can wait in a tizzy, wringing your hands, or you can accept it.

Dr. Alan Berger told a support group, "Sometimes you have to lower your expectations." They were in shock. "What? You mean give in to the pain? You're saying I should not fight back?"

"Yes," he said. "Just tell yourself, 'This is a crummy day, but things will be better tomorrow.'"

Many have been brought up to believe they must hang tough, they must fight back, they must muscle through the pain. Dr. Berger says "Relax. Take a break." Sure enough, people in my support group discovered that they rebounded more quickly than if they had gritted their teeth and finished the day with their chores all checked off. If you carry on with the discomfort, the following day you may be exhausted. The pain goes faster if you do less on your schedule and leave the rest for mañana. Barbara M. didn't buy it. "I could never do that," she said. "I have too much to do." I am hopeful she will eventually come around.

- Sometimes you have to lower your expectations. The pain goes away more quickly than if you muscle through it.

Laughing: The Art and Science

There's a wonderful cartoon from an old *New Yorker* magazine that shows a huge porcupine staring at a gigantic unclassifiable dog with dozens of quills in his nose. The pooch says, "On the plus side, you've cured my back pain." Diversion is everything. And a good laugh is especially diverting.

Beth Cole is "a certified laugh leader," which she tells me while giggling. She says 300 "laughologists" inhabit the United States, all of whom have gone to workshops. Laughter is a great mood interrupter, if you are stuck in the doldrums.

Beth starts people laughing just for the sake of laughing. She might say to them, "Say 'ALO-HA' to your neighbor and then say 'ALO-Ha-Ha-Ha' and so on." And pretty soon the whole room is laughing. There's a bank of 150 of such exercises or games on her website.

- Laughter reduces pain. Articles have been written about it. "Laughter brings about happiness. You don't have to be happy to laugh," says Beth Cole.

- Cole says there hasn't been a lot of definitive research on the laughter–pain connection; most of it is anecdotal. "People say laughing improves their health and eases their pain. It certainly takes your mind off it."

- Visit www.worldlaughtertour.org if you are interested in learning more.

In 1964, Norman Cousins was felled by ankylosing spondylitis, a condition in which connective tissue in the spine disintegrates. But his death did not occur until he'd fought a remarkable fight. When his doctor virtually gave up, Cousins took things into his own hands and found that funny shows, especially TV's *Candid Camera*, and Marx Brothers movies, made him laugh. His landmark book, *Anatomy of an Illness*, let the world take a serious look at the relationship between laughter and illness. The book also described his recovery, as well as his thoughts on medicine and the patient's responsibility. Cousins lived a good life and died 26 years after his initial diagnosis.

- Beth Cole says, "Three things happen when you laugh: Your anger dissolves, you stop focusing on your illness or problem, and you stop looking inward."

- The first Sunday in May is designated as World Laughter Day, but don't wait till then to laugh. Be a clown.

You have a choice as to how people see you, and it'll make you feel better if they see you as "upbeat," rather than "sorrowful." Some people thrive on "pity parties," which isn't healthful or helpful for anyone. They go through life as the doleful donkey Eeyore in Winnie-the-Pooh. *You might say, Who cares what people think?* That's a self-assured way to feel, but that's not the point. It's how you see yourself that matters, and if you see yourself as an upbeat, positive person, doing OK, you will be. Laughter is not fattening, and it costs nothing. It is a human being's way of wagging a tail. People prefer a funny person over a drama queen any day. And you get fewer wrinkles if you smile than if you frown.

Some people with chronic ailments use laughter as a smokescreen. They need to disguise how they feel, and that works in their favor. Ian W. was stricken with neuropathy from the neck down at age 19, but managed to claw his way back to a fairly normal existence. He was always cheerful and had a good sense of humor. People said there couldn't be much wrong with him because he was always happy. Was he denying his pain? No. Was he living a lie? No. His good-natured attitude prevented people from feeling sorry for him, so he invented a cheerful attitude and it made him feel energized, and even normal.

- An amusing DVD is *The Joy of Stress*.[19] Loretta LaRoche is a stand-up comedienne who talks about stress in a way you may never have heard before. She is a nationally known lecturer on stress management and founded The Humor Potential, Inc. In addition, she is a faculty member for The Behavior Institute of Medicine, an affiliate of Harvard Medical School. One of her mantras: STOP GLOBAL WHINING!

- If you want to prevent "Hardening of the Attitude," LaRoche says you need to stop "awfulizing." This jolly-ologist reminds us that we are Driving the Bus. Our attitude is in our hands. And, she says, how your face looks (sad, happy, grim) makes you feel a certain way. Dump your misery gene and laugh every day.

- Lighten up, and you'll be enlightened, comedian Mike Myers says, in his more serious moments.

Loving the Sun You're In

My friend Ann P.'s granddaughter Gina told her, "Grandma, you have curly skin." So use that phrase if someone points out your wrinkles. *It's just curly skin. That's all.* And let's rejoice: Wrinkles aren't painful.

Getting a little sun is important (the vitamin D factor), but tanning must be done carefully if you have peripheral neuropathy. Neuropathy that includes numbness in your legs or hands may prevent you from knowing you are burning. That's why, if you have peripheral neuropathy, you have to be particularly vigilant.

- Even with the best sunscreen, don't stay out in the sun too long. Early in the morning and later in the afternoon is best: before 10:00 A.M. and after 4:00 P.M.

- Choose your protection according to your skin color. Children, people with very fair skin, those who live in high altitudes or in the southern states, or anyone who has had skin cancer should be extra cautious and use a lotion with protection against the two types of ultraviolet (UV) rays: UVA (Think A for Age: they make you age faster) and UVB (Think B for Burn: they make you burn faster). A dermatologist came up with that.

- Be sure to get a skin check once a year (or more often if you are in a high-risk category) by a professional; between times, examine your skin frequently.

- Don't even think about using sunlamps or tanning beds. The beds send out UVA and UVB rays. Once again, if your skin has less sensitivity due to numbness, it can be seriously damaged.

- Clothing that protects your skin from harmful rays is available. It is fairly expensive; however, it works well.

- To help avoid cataracts, wear sunglasses. UV light is a primary cause of cataracts, as is advancing age.

- Consult your local newspaper. Many list the UV Index, which tells you on a scale of 0–10 how high the power of the sun's rays will be for that day. The higher the number, the greater your chances for burning.

- The opposite side of the coin is that, yes, we need some sun to get enough vitamin D, the sunshine vitamin. Read Drs. Oz's and Roizen's chapter called, "Major Ager: UV Radiation—How the Sun Can Nourish or Destroy Your Body" in *You: Staying Young*.[6] It's an in-depth look at this good sun/bad sun issue.

Medical Supply Stores

Don't underestimate the value of medical supply stores. Bob W. found something to twist the key in his car's ignition more easily. The motor nerves that control his wrist muscles were causing a problem until he found a 2-inch-wide plastic cover that fits over the key handle. Before you zoom past a supply store, stop and see how they can help you. You might find something to assist you with putting on clothes or shoes, or doing other everyday tasks that might be difficult because of peripheral neuropathy. If they don't have an item you want, many stores can order it for you from their catalog. Inventories vary by store, so check out all the stores near you.

Meditation

To meditate is to listen with a receptive heart.
—BUDDHA

Neuropathy is not a "been there, done that" affliction. Your symptoms may wax and wane, but the nerve problem will "stick it," just as a gymnast doing a round-off back handspring must stick it at the finish. Your peripheral neuropathy will probably be with you until a cure comes along. That's why a quiet mind that cleaves to meditation must become your goal.

So much has been written on meditation. You may or may not be interested in pursuing it. Dip into one of the countless books on the subject. Delve into industrial-strength theories behind the fascinating history of meditation, or read more user-friendly memoirs written by people who have discovered meditation. Consider *Eat, Pray, Love*, by Elizabeth Gilbert.[20] It was a huge bestseller, but it seems that people either adored it or couldn't read it. It's an account of her life following divorce and her travels in search of peace.

- Amy Gross, former editor-in-chief of Oprah's Magazine, *O*, is a practicing Buddhist and a believer in meditation, practicing Vipassana insight meditation. Meditation is done in silence, and silence, she says, is medicine. A therapist friend of hers gave her a sign saying, "My remedy for everything is to be quiet." She feels silence becomes more valuable as we get older.

- Meditation is as easy as finding a comfortable place in which to sit or lie down, turning off the phone or TV, and breathing slowly with your eyes shut. Breathe deeply and focus on your breathing. One to five minutes is all it takes, and you can do it several times a day.

- If nothing else, breathe. So many people with neuropathy are so uptight, strung out, and in a tizzy that I want to take hold of them and say, "Stop! Just breathe. Count to ten. Calm down. Don't make a catastrophe out of this." (See the section on breathing in Chapter 3.)

- Meditation has helped people for thousands of years. Why should it be any different for you?

Napping Is My Favorite Sport

I found my niche early in life. My first report card in kindergarten announced, "Marguerite is a good rester." Terrific. Forget about arithmetic, spelling, reading . . . Let the kid rest! Call me the original Power Rester.

Recently, I read an article about a man with neuropathy who uses a comfy recliner as his "nappy chair." Kind of the reverse of a "time-out chair." Some say they can't nap in the middle of the day. Others love to re-energize themselves with a power nap. I have heard, however, that sumo wrestlers nap after lunch because sleeping after their noon chow is the best way to bulk up. Oh dear . . . .

The Harvard School of Public Health completed a research program with 24,000 people and concluded that you are 40% less likely to die from heart problems if you are an afternoon napper.[21] All you need are 10–20 minutes after lunch, and you will feel more energetic and productive the rest of the day. Run this one by your boss.

In an article in the 2002 *Neuropathy News*, Dr. Scott Berman, a man after my own heart—a chronic napper who wants to turn napping into an Olympic sport—states that according to a study by Merkes and colleagues, fatigue is one of the three things that annoy PNers the most.[22] Fatigue was noted in more than 80% of the people in the study. So don't feel guilty; if you are tired, snooze. Don't you love that word? Snoooooooooooze. I'll get back to work on this in a little while. . . .

Pain Management

Alan Berger, MD, elaborated on the subject of pain and attitude in my 2002 book, *If You're Having a Crummy Day, Brush Off the Crumbs*:[23]

"Pain is one of the most common and disabling manifestations of peripheral neuropathy. It has been my experience that patients' ability to function despite pain, is in large part dependent on their attitude.

"Why is it that some people refuse to allow even severe pain to disable them while others, with less discomfort, are completely incapacitated?

"In many ways, the ... difference among those who cope with pain and those who don't is what they choose to focus on. Fortunately, the object of one's focus is under free will, although it may take great willpower and mental training. Functioning patients think, '*I know I have pain, and it's bothersome, but I need to concentrate on what I intend to do today and not let the pain interfere.*' Those who cannot function tend to think, 'Oh God, another day of pain. I can't take it.'

"The key is choosing what you focus on and finding what you want to be the dominant focus of your life. Some people do it naturally, and they tend to be productive and happy. Others have to train their brains to change their focus ....

"A patient's attitude goes a long way in determining how well he or she copes. Those who accept their condition and their limitations are better able to function than those who continually feel victimized. The bitterness associated with being the victim appears to exacerbate the pain, preventing the patient from being fully functional."

Prescription for Wellness: A Wagging Tail

Money will buy a pretty good dog, but it won't buy the wag of his tail.
—JOSH BILLINGS

No matter how much cats fight, there always seem to be plenty of kittens.
—ABRAHAM LINCOLN

Go right ahead and skip this section if you do not like dogs and cats or are allergic to them; however, if you think you might want one in your house, read on. There's an important reason to consider a furry pal.

As you know, it is very common for people with neuropathy to become depressed. Taking a pill for depression, along with your pain meds, can sometimes result in a difficult cocktail for your system. A pet might just be better for you than an antidepressant pill. When my dog, Lily, is happy, which is practically all the time judging by her flapping tail, I am never in the dumps. A dog knows the ultimate happiness is to enjoy life, and they will love life if they are owned by a loving person.

In the morning, when Sweetie and Precious are lying near Julie P., taking up residence on pillows between her and her husband, she knows her day will begin with sunshine, no matter how her feet feel and even if it's pouring cats and dogs.

As so many do, she fostered two abandoned dogs from a shelter to help them become social critters, and then couldn't bear to part with them. In the beginning, she didn't think about the value of her dachshunds to her neuropathy. Then she realized how wonderful it was that they insisted on their morning walk, a great benefit to her.

A recent newspaper article talked about the therapeutic value of other animals, too: birds, rabbits, miniature horses, and llamas. I'm not ready to nestle in bed with a llama, but thanks anyway. Pet Denver Partners and the American Humane Association have noted a groundswell of interest in the human–animal bond. They predict pet therapy will become an integral part of how illnesses will be treated in the future.

Lisa Pollard, CEO and founder of Actions Dog Training in Jacksonville, Florida, has been able to "read" dogs since the age of ten, when she brought up a Keeshond and the dog's two litters. She's been in the dog training business for 30 years. "Dogs will get you walking," she says. "If you are having a bad patch, they will understand if you cut their walk short. Dogs sense when you're not well." How comforting is that? If you're not sure if a dog or cat is really right for you, try fostering. Your local animal shelter has lots of animals that need a home in which to stay until they find their "forever home." The great thing about fostering is that it's a trial run. If you happen to fall in love with a little furry bundle, you can keep it; if not, the pet you fostered will find a home elsewhere.

- Choose a dog with a somewhat low energy level if your neuropathy precludes you from walking fast. A calmer dog might be perfect if you need to stop in place to steady yourself and re-balance.

- Watching the silly antics of a kitten chasing after birdie toys or a puppy trying to capture a laser light is hilarious and can get you laughing, which is always good for what hurts.

- Divert the discomfort of hand or foot pain by stroking a furry pet. The spring 2008 issue of *All Animals*, a magazine of the Humane Society of the United States (HSUS), says that Americans own 88 million cats and 74 million dogs.[24]

- Talk to a shelter about fostering or adopting. Every year 4 to 5 million dogs and cats are placed in homes, according to HSUS. And 25% of the dogs in shelters are purebred according to HSUS.

- An older dog that has been housebroken and isn't eating pens, pencils, or gnawing on the legs of your cherrywood dining room table (thanks a lot, Lily) might be easier for senior citizens to care for. A more sedate older cat is another good option.

- Pollard says, "Dogs are a reason for people to think about something else besides their pain." She adds, "Dogs are huge lickers, and if you feel your feet or hands would enjoy a good bath, a dog's lapping tongue would be a great side benefit to having a dog."

- Pets for the Elderly Foundation pays up to $50 toward the adoption fee if you adopt a pet from one of 58 animal shelters in 31 states. Call 866-849-3598 or visit www.petsfortheelderly.org for more information. Many shelters offer adoption discounts to elders.[25] Older citizens in particular should consider adopting an older dog that's already gone through the difficult puppy years.

- Leona Shedden, executive director of the Jacksonville Humane Society, told me recently that all shelters supported by Purina as their corporate food sponsor have a program in place called Pets For People. She said, "The program is for seniors 60 years and older. If a pet is 6 years or older, seniors can get the pet for free. Our shelter—and most others—work hard to find the right pet to match the right person and his or her energy level and lifestyle."

Physical Therapy

Brian Gupton, a physical therapist at Ponte Vedra Physical Therapy, Inc. in Ponte Vedra Beach, Florida, says that in the last 2 years more people who have peripheral neuropathy have been coming to his facility for physical therapy. "Often they come because they can't tolerate the various pain medications, so physicians are encouraging them to try PT." Gupton says a therapist can help people with peripheral neuropathy who have issues with range of motion, mobility, flexibility, muscle weakness, atrophy, dizziness, loss of coordination, balance, and other problems. An expert physical therapist will be knowledgeable in all these things. Therapists can also apply massage, ultrasound, and electrical stimulation. "One of the first things that improves is circulation," Gupton says.

Unconsciously or consciously, you may be compensating for your pain by walking, standing, and sitting incorrectly. This will serve only to further deteriorate your body. Proper exercise or PT can help you. Working through the pain will not. Eugene Richardson, Neuropathy Association support group leader and neuropathy advocate, says, "Damaged motor and sensory nerves can become worse when they are pushed beyond a certain point. You must constantly monitor your program. Work according to how you feel at the time of the therapy or exercise. Do not work through the pain!"

People in a support group might help you find a PT program or therapist that you will like. In some instances, doctor-referred therapy is covered by insurance programs, but some cover only a limited number of sessions.

Reflexology

In the interest of research for this book, I forced myself to go to a spa one day and try out reflexology. What a trouper. This was not the hardest work regarding *Cope*. Trust me. I was in Connecticut on vacation, and an article in a local paper guided my hand to the telephone where I made an appointment at Aetheria, a day spa, in New Canaan.

Alisa Arakelian, a trained certified reflexologist, cushioned me with soft pillows and proceeded to let her gentle hands and soothing cream work their wonders on my feet. She told me archeologists found art carvings of people massaging feet on a tomb in Saqqara, Egypt, dating back to 2330 B.C. Arakelian said reflexology is a healing art that can relieve but does not cure. It works well with allergies, headaches, arthritis, and a lot more. "I have had amazing results," she said. "People can get into a deep state of relaxation." I was taking notes; it wasn't quite so relaxing as it might be for you.

Reflexologists thumb-walk on your feet and sometimes hands. Particular spots on the feet and hands are connected to corresponding places in the body: the liver, the head, the back, heart, and uterus. Arakelian proceeded to say how the feet are mapped to correlate to the rest of the body. If you get a massage on those big toes of yours, for instance, you might feel relief from headache. Arakelian said she can identify problems such as migraines or swelling in the gall bladder or liver. "You will sleep better tonight," she tells me. Yes, I did, perhaps because I babysat for my three grandkids later in the day.

"Your feet are your foundation," Arakelian continued. "Picture a tissue box, then put a crooked one on top of that, and another crooked one on top of that one and keep going. The whole thing will be off balance."

The foot massage was pleasant and enjoyable. As with all these healing methods, you have to have the right frame of mind and help it along by believing in it.

- If you like to try anything once, try reflexology. You may be surprised at how great your feet feel, but you do need to keep going back for longer-lasting results. It's bound to help your blood circulation, at least for a little while.

Reiki

Lynn Davis Slavin, Registered Master Teacher and member of the International Association of Reiki Practitioners, sees patients in her home in Darien, Connecticut.

If you are not familiar with this form of massage, visit her site at www.wellnessmattersllc.com to learn more. A genuine, likeable soul, and someone who has performed Reiki on me, she provides us with these tips:

- "When used on patients suffering from neuropathy, I have found, during a Reiki session, which lasts about 50 or 60 minutes, that people are able to tune out the discomfort and experience a cessation of pain."

- "In almost every case of clients with neuropathy in their hands and/or feet, I am able to feel an enormous amount of energy 'buzzing' or flowing in areas that cause people pain. This indicates that energy is being stimulated, blockages are released, and a healthier balance is created in the body. Clients say, 'I am more in control of my symptoms.'"

- "Reiki is cumulative; therefore, the more Reiki sessions, the deeper the healing. Everything that helps control symptoms has a place in an individual's health care plan."

Relax

In 1975, Herbert Benson's ground-breaking book, *The Relaxation Response*,[26] struck a chord with millions. He simplified what people felt was mumbo jumbo of the mystics. The book is just as valuable today. Let it resonate with you. Your heart rate may go down and the calm might help your peripheral neuropathy.

Seasonal Affective Disorder: Summer or Winter

The winter season takes away sunlight at an early hour in the afternoon, which has a serious negative impact on many people. This can affect how they feel mentally as well as physically. Michael Terman, director of New York-Presbyterian Hospital's Center for Light Treatment and Biological Rhythms, calls seasonal affective disorder (SAD) a significant medical problem that can disable people.[27] He says we can feel tired when we waken due to sunlight getting to us later in the morning. That dragged-out feeling can last all day long. And then it darkens earlier, giving us overall fewer hours of sunlight.

When you have neuropathy, SAD symptoms can worsen. The change in the amount of daylight puts a kink in your body clock. You feel out of sorts, out of sync. You may feel less cheerful, less productive.

Conversely, some PNers say they have a hard time getting through summer. They, too, have SAD, just at a different time of year. Denise W. says the heat aggravates her symptoms. She is bothered by intense sunlight.

And, while heat bothers some people with peripheral neuropathy, the winter chill bothers others; extremes in temperature can make PNers feel their personal body thermostat is out of whack.

If it's obvious that you're in a downward spiral because of the weather, don't wait in a tizzy until the weather changes. Try these tips, collected from support groups and The Neuropathy Association's *Neuropathy E-News*® online newsletter:

- Let go. Take a deep breath, and don't fight the weather. Flow with it.

- If winter's your enemy, be sure to get outside, even if it's only for 10 minutes a day. You will feel sunnier after a sun bath.

- A light therapy box uses strong rays of light to trick you into thinking it is summer. Take a chance on a light box and see if it works.

- If the summer heat bothers you, take up pool aerobics in the morning to feel cooler early in the day, or go to a pool for a refreshing dunk.

- Summer, winter—all year around—you mustn't stop exercising, even though the weather gets you down. Exercise gets the blood moving, and your oxygen levels and the hormones that influence your mood—your endorphins—will flow better and you'll feel more chipper. Staying active is vital not just for physical health, but for emotional and mental health too.

- See friends and family. Becoming a hermit is not a good idea. If your family lives in another state, remember the phrase, "Friends are family we choose for ourselves." This is especially important if you live on your own.

- Up north, it's common to get cabin fever in the winter. In the south, you can also get that locked-in feeling if the sun wipes you out so much that you have to stay indoors. Plan your outings to coincide with the sun: In the dead heat of summer in the south, get out early and be back well before noon or wait till late. In the north in winter, give the landscape a chance to thaw and plan excursions when the sun is working harder.

- North or south, try to check out something new: a museum you've never been to, an art gallery, a cultural center. Maybe take a course.

- Not only *see*, but *do* something different. If you've never painted, try it. Read a play with friends, have an indoor picnic. Become creative. Become imaginative.

- What do you love to do? Dine out? Go to a movie? Make a date night with a friend or spouse and go see a play.

Self-hypnosis

Self-hypnosis was the topic of a lecture at the Northern California Chapter of The Neuropathy Association, May 1, 2008. The speaker was Jay Tinsman, MD, licensed Marriage and Family Therapist in Sacramento California. Bev Anderson, Northern California Chapter of The Neuropathy Association leader, was kind enough to send me her notes following his talk.

Tinsman's 2-2-2 Training Method

- I give myself permission to relax about all my problems with my pain. I accept my pain without surrendering to it.
- I'm allowing my perception of pain to fade into the background more often.
- I'm narrowing the constant thoughts I have about my pain, and I am worrying less frequently.
- I'm letting go of my fear and worry of both present and possible future pain.
- I am keeping a cool head and allowing myself to substitute more pleasant sensations for what I now experience as pain.
- I am becoming more sensitive to the details of my pain, and I realize much of what I feel is not pain at all, but some other sensation. (OR) I am becoming less sensitive to the details of my pain because my mind is occupied with more interesting things.
- I am allowing my mind and body to learn to develop pain relief in the affected area.
- I have resolved to ignore my pain and start enjoying life again.
- I am doing everything appropriate to lessen my pain.
- I am allowing my subconscious mind to do whatever it needs to do to let me experience relief and I don't need to know the details.
- Pain is my friend because it reminds me I am alive and it protects me from harm. That part I will keep and I will let go of the rest.

Reprinted with permission from Jay Tinsman, MA, Sacramento, California. Web site: www.jaytinsmanma.com.

The main thrust of his speech was that we have a mind–body connection that can be tapped, and we can summon our inner resources to override pain.

You need to be determined to do this, and you must persevere. Practice it and figure out what works. You must not dwell on your past pain or worry about future pain. The best thing is to take 30 minutes a day and slow your natural force against the pain to develop well-being. Words are the most powerful tools we have. They can develop and they can destroy. Hypnosis consists of using specific words to guide us to the subconscious.

Jay Tinsman sent me his notes for this same lecture in an e-mail. He wrote, "Our minds and thoughts can influence our body in specific ways. We can find comfort even when our nerve endings are telling us something else."

Here is his "2-2-2 Training" method:

- Find a spot where you are least likely to be disturbed. Tell yourself why you are doing what you are about to do (to alleviate your pain) and then take a deep breath, close your eyes, and say, "Relax."

- Go to a quiet place in your mind where you can relax physically and mentally for 2 minutes.

- After you have done that, open your eyes and look at a few of the subconscious suggestions listed in the accompanying box for 2 minutes.

- Concentrate on your favorite topics. Say them aloud, quietly. Then take a deep breath and bring your mind to a state of relaxation for 2 minutes.

That's it. You can do this once a day, several times a day, or as often as you like.

Self-Talk: Watch Your Language

Sometime in the late 1960s, Jean Neiditch, founder of Weight Watchers, spoke to a large audience of women in New York City at the time when her program was taking off around the country. "Ladies," she said, "Do not use the word 'disaster' when you are talking about eating a piece of chocolate cake. A disaster is when a tornado destroys your house or a loved one is hit by a car."

People often use the word "disaster" for small stuff. My mother used to holler, "Don't say that!" if I'd tell her I'd gotten a disastrous grade in math. Good advice. And there's another reason to watch your language: It doesn't do you any good to talk mean to yourself. Do you talk negatively about yourself? You might say:

- "This stupid neuropathy is just ruining my life." Or ....

- "I'm so stupid. I can't (fill in the blank) any more."

- "I'm really a dope when it comes to ...."

My daughter, who is quite self-confident and has a healthy amount of self-esteem, once said to me, when I gave her a specially nice present, "Oh wow, Mom. I am not worthy." She had started to say it all the time. I told her to stop. "If you say you are not worthy, you will feel not worthy. And that is negative self-talk. You are worthy!" (When my son proofread this book, he wanted to know how come his sister got a "specially nice present" and what exactly was it anyway?)

- Be careful how you talk about yourself. Negative thoughts can sink you. Speak nicely about yourself to yourself and to others. Love yourself, and you can love others.

Someone I knew in grade school has been debilitated because of neuropathy (and other ailments) and bedridden for years. When she calls, she never asks how I am, how my family is, or anything about my life. All she talks about is herself, and the conversation is negative from start to finish: her husband, her children, and, of course, her health. Other people who know her say it takes them an hour before they can get off the phone.

Being bedridden has got to be tremendously frustrating, and I feel deeply compassionate toward her, but I do think she could find something to enjoy. "What do you do all day," I asked. "Oh," she said, "it's too painful to do anything." She used to be a straight-A student. No crossword puzzles? No books? No educational videos? She has made her bed and climbed in. Period. Nobody has to live that way, and you get the feeling that she doesn't want any suggestions to make her life more pleasant.

- For every day you stay in bed, it takes one day to mend. (That's what my mom told me.) Get up. Get dressed. If you can, walk a little every day, and then a little more each day.

Singing in the Sunshine: Laughing in the Rain

During the 1970s, living through the brutal winters of New England, I made a commitment to sing with the Stamford Masterworks Chorale, and went to rehearsal every Monday night. Often I was exhausted and didn't feel like rehearsing, but it acted as therapy, and I always returned home relaxed and happy, even when we sang industrial-strength requiems.

More or less, I've sung in a group ever since that time. For me, it's a tonic. I sing with Singers By The Sea, in Jacksonville Beach, Florida, a lovable and funny group of seniors. We sing more or less 18 times a year at nursing homes and retirement villages. The chorus members are in their 50s and older, so you can be sure many of us have plenty of ailments, but that's the last thing on our minds. And we don't sweat missing a few notes in a tricky score of *Moon River* either. Peripheral neuropathy teaches you not to sweat the small stuff.

In the March/April issue of *Arthritis Today*, Francine Kaplan[28] tells of the benefits of expanding your lungs. Many people say that when they sing, they forget their pain.

- Studies by Harvard and Yale say chorale singing boosts your immune system.[28]

- A study at Temple University in the Arts and Quality of Life Research Center found many benefits of music with regard to chronic pain.[28]

- Look around for a group with whom you might be compatible. If you can blend in nicely and can read the notation (or stand next to someone who can help you out), you might be an asset to the group, and singing can definitely help alleviate your pain.

- *The British Journal of Nursing* reported that anxiety and depression lessen with singing therapy (especially following surgery).[29] There are even vocal psychotherapists.

Spas, Hot Tubs, Jacuzzis

Unlike using extremely cold water, which can be damaging to your nerves, you may use saunas, hot tubs, Jacuzzis, etc., unless you have autonomic neuropathy, in which case the heat can dangerously lower your blood pressure. Also, you will not cause nerve damage if you use a hot pad as long as it's on a low or medium heat setting. These are OK from a neuropathic standpoint, with a couple of warnings:

- If you have sensory neuropathy, your skin may not be able to recognize when the water is too hot, so proceed with caution and don't scald yourself. The common wisdom is that, if you enjoy spas, use them. It's like getting massages: Some people don't like them; others swear by them.

- Be careful getting in and out of hot tubs if you have balance difficulties.

Spirituality

*If we know so little about the medical, physical realm of life,
why should we be surprised that there are mysteries in the
spiritual world? Life is an unlimited sea of mysteries.
There are no easy answers. Don't look for them.*
—Pastor John Dolaghan, The Chapel at Sawgrass, Ponte Vedra Beach, Florida

Alice Walker, author of *The Color Purple*, said you don't need to belong to an organized religion to feel a connection with the universe. Connecting with one's spirit doesn't mean you have to go to church. People connect through their various circles of life. If you are an actor, you feel connected with your fellow thespians. If you take a class, there's a commonality with other students, and so on. People in the same boat, with the same feelings of frustration, can gain solace and support from one another. Communication opens up, and they do not feel so alone; they feel linked to one another.

David N. Elkins, clinical psychologist and professor of psychology at Pepperdine University, says spiritual growth is not about organized religion; it is about becoming one with the wonder of life.[30] Nature and almost anything that resonates to our very depths are sources of soul nurturing.

Life's wonders can be found in ordinary things. Find the extraordinary in everyday things. Be amazed at a perfectly formed rose, a melody that makes your heart soar, a lake that shimmers like a jewel. Savor your days of wellness. And never feel you have to defend or explain your feelings of spirituality to those who don't understand, maybe even to people in your own family. Spirituality is in large part being aware of others' worries and fears and helping them feel less lost, less alone.

Your gratitude journal, which is really just another way of counting your blessings, is an outward expression of your inward joyousness. Spirituality is your private garden of joy to go to any time you want.

There's a wonderful phrase that I wrote down a year or so ago, unfortunately without noting the author. It goes like this: "I never feel so accompanied as when I am alone, and I have figured it out. It is because God is always beside me."

- Subscribe to a daily devotional guide and enjoy meditations every day, or perhaps a book of daily meditations that fit your needs would suffice.

- You can be as spiritual as you want to be.

Stress

Stress is everywhere, and it's making us sick and unhealthy. That is not to say our neuropathy is caused by stress, but it sure doesn't help it. The American Psychological Association found, in a 2007 project, that for most of us, the prime sources of stress are money and work; 33% say they are living with great stress; 48% feel their stress has increased over the past 5 years.[31] Stress, good or bad, usually makes neuropathy worse. And think of the worry lines and wrinkles you avoid when you stress less.

Saying to people who are stressed, "Don't worry about it," or "Stop stressing," simply doesn't work. "Chill out" may really make them mad. Bottom line: To control stress, you have to make conscious changes in your life—that stressed, burned-out feeling can happen after months of working too hard or dealing with difficult relationships.

- If you are constantly exhausted, or feel overwhelmed or anxious, don't let yourself adapt to those emotional barriers to happiness. Do something about it. Depending on what your angst is, you may need to plan to do certain things. If you're exhausted, eating a hot fudge sundae isn't going to help; a nap is what you need. When he is upset, Bill D. focuses on exercise. Betty D. takes anger or stress out on her silverware and polishes like crazy, and Lilly gardens or cooks.

- Stress-proof your days by analyzing what you do. If you can eliminate things, such as ironing, let it go. Delegate household chores. Make up a chart.

- Plan on time for yourself. Instead of doing your tasks by starting with things you don't like doing, start with the fun stuff. It might put you in a good mood, so that you sail through the rest of the chores more easily.

- Do something to soothe and relax yourself. Take a hot bath in winter, a cool one in summer.

The Cure Within: A History of Mind-Body Medicine, by Anne Harrington,[32] delves into a good deal of research on the subject of stress which was, in the 1950s and 1960s, shown to have a major impact on our health. In her chapter called "Broken by Modern Life," she says it was in the 1970s that researchers realized it wasn't so much what the stress was, but rather how you handled it. The mind has a lot to do with how we cope with stress. Harrington calls it "creative coping," and we humans have a tremendous capacity for being creative in this area.

Tigger or Eeyore?

Randy Pausch, a professor at Carnegie Mellon, talked on various TV programs during the fall of 2007 and gained the admiration of people around the world. His battle with pancreatic cancer was documented on YouTube and in periodicals. His book, *The Last Lecture*,[33] flew off store bookshelves each time he appeared on television specials such as *Primetime*. Pausch told us how he was dealing with the difficulties of dying, with life all around him. Do you remember when Diane Sawyer asked him if he was in any pain? His answer was, yes, his neuropathy. He died on July 25, 2008, at the age of 47. A brilliant teacher, communicator, and humorist, he handled his illness with about as much grace, wit, and courage as any person can. He was married with three young children and people who knew his story were captivated by him.

- Pausch said one can go through life as the Winnie the Pooh character Tigger—always optimistic and full of spit and vinegar, or as Eeyore—doleful, pessimistic, constantly worrying about life's gloomy, gray days. You Tiggers out there will find much meaning in this book. I hope the Eeyores will give it a chance as well.

Recapture Your Childlike Love for Flowers and Nature

Yesterday I received in the mail a children's book to review titled *Some Helpful Tips for a Better World and a Happier Life*, by Rebecca Doughty.[34] I've lost count of exactly how many books I reviewed, but it's around 1,600 or so. It amused me that I am writing a book on tips, and this appears on my doorstep from a publisher. The cover tells me it's a book "for all ages," which is true, more or less.

One tip for happiness that works for any age (and for the ages) is to "smell the roses." When my dog died in 2007, one of the things I missed most was taking him out several times a day for his "performance." I hadn't realized how much I counted on those trips to settle me into a cheerful mood. Charlie and I would check out our little corner of the universe and drink it in. How easy to fill up a gratitude journal by reveling in the sunshine, marveling at a good soaking rain, or watching the antics of the wildlife on a lake. Nature is bliss.

Toxic People

Dealing with a chronic illness can seem like a full-time job, and if you are around toxic people, your misery will be compounded. Here's a challenge, if you dare to accept it: Don't do toxic. Don't go there. Dump the whole enchiladaville of anything toxic—whether it's people or chemicals in food, shampoos, or cleaning supplies. Toxic whatever can grow all around you and smother you like a kudzu vine. People in Thailand say *mai pen lai*, which means "let it go." Forget about it. Drop it. Say, "Never mind."

- Toxic people harm anybody's health, but people who are in pain need to focus their energy toward people who bring out the best in them. Being around people laden with anger or negativity harms you. It's similar to being around smokers, passively inhaling their smoke. In short: Banish toxic people, control freaks, and the like.

Sometimes we think we can help them. But they are not going to change.

Judith Orloff's *Positive Energy: 10 Extraordinary Prescriptions for Transforming Fatigue, Stress & Fear Into Vibrance, Strength, & Love* helps us understand toxicity.[35]

One of Orloff's important chapters is "Protect Yourself from Energy Vampires." We have all been exposed to them: people who sap you of your good humor. They take from you more than you give, leaving you feeling sad or empty. Their negativity casts a dark and gloomy spell over everybody. It robs people of an inner sunshine.

She labels Energy Vampires this way: The Sob Sister or whiner: she feels she is a victim. The Blamer: he makes you feel as if it's your fault that he is so beleaguered. The Drama Queen: she tends to catastrophize and gets hysterical over little things. The Fixer-Upper: he hands over his life problems and wants you to repair them. She mentions other categories, but you get the idea.

- Your neuropathy needs your attention, not a difficult, toxic relative or spouse. A friend who is toxic is easier to shed, but if that someone is a relative or living in your house, especially if they are verbally or physically abusive, don't tolerate it. You need help—a pastor, close friend, or support group.

Years ago, someone stunned and angered me with a senseless act of meanness. (No, it wasn't a marital issue.) I am usually good at shaking off anger, but this also involved disbelief, sadness, betrayal, and a host of other negative emotions that left me riddled with emotional pain. It dismayed me that anyone could be that hurtful. My daughter said, "Mom, just put him in a blender." She made me laugh for the first time in weeks. Another way of thinking is: "Don't let them rent space in your head," a delightful sentence courtesy of a dog park friend, Madelyn L.

We have all known mean-spirited people. Keynote presenter Cammy Dierking at a *Speaking of Women's Health* conference in August 2008 calls them "emotional vampires." They can rub off on you if you let them. And, more than you think, you rub off on other people, too. "Never underestimate how you affect others," said Simon Bailey, author of *Release Your Brilliance*, at the book festival,[36] *Much Ado About Books*, in Jacksonville, Florida.

When unkind, narrow-minded, intolerant people aim their barbs at you, they may appear to be happy some of the time, but they don't deserve it. Victor Hugo said, "To be perfectly happy, it does not suffice to possess happiness; it is necessary to have deserved it."

Orloff recommends that you breathe differently when you are in the presence of an Energy Vampire. Let your breath function like a "vacuum cleaner."

Suction back every ounce of energy he has sucked away from you and keep doing this. She says if you feel tense or on guard around a person, or if you feel put down and are feeling negative vibrations, step away. Around positive people, you will intuitively feel relaxed, calm, safe. They almost give off a radiance, and you feel a sense of compassion, hope. In short, they make you feel better. Isn't this feeling of wellness what we're all trying to find?

- Don't let negative people suck the life out of you.

- Nurture yourself when you are not feeling well by surrounding yourself with optimistic people who give off positive energy.

- When your neuropathy leaves you feeling dreary, it's easier to be happy if you meditate or pray, and prayer is gratitude for being alive.

Tweak Your Wellness Plan

- Plan ahead for those times when you can't focus on anything but your pain. You can. You need a bunch of ideas to divert you. A movie works for some, shopping with a friend works for others. My personal favorite is Howard E.'s plan of attack: "Sit in front of the fridge with the door open and a knife and fork in your hands."

- Always get up, get dressed, and, for women, get out lipstick and mascara. A bit of perfume is nice, too. When you hurt, slopping around in a bathrobe until noon or later can become a bad habit.

- Read passages from your religion's scriptures regularly if you have made friends with that book, and maybe even if you haven't. If you let it, scripture can tell you a lot about how to cope with your pains from neuropathy.

- Volunteer. If you are helpful to somebody or can be a good steward for an organization, you will go home feeling better. Speaking of which . . . next topic, please.

Volunteering: Be Good Bone-Deep

Doing good is the greatest happiness.
—OLD CHINESE PROVERB

If you are having a day that is "just not fair," allow yourself 5 minutes to commiserate with someone—or have your own personal five-star, world-class pity party. And forget about "not fair." Everybody has some medical ailment or other worry to gripe about. After you've been a grouch for 5 minutes, tell yourself,

"That's enough." All right, take 10 minutes. Now, here's what you do when time's up (trumpets and flourishes): Get involved with something greater than yourself. And that means *volunteer*.

If anyone can tell you about the virtues of volunteering, Irene Beer certainly can. For 11 years, she has had intravenous immunoglobulin (IVIg) infusion treatments on a regular basis, and has never stopped volunteering for The Neuropathy Association or leading support groups. She considers volunteering one of the best coping mechanisms for people with any chronic disease.

Dr. Gerson Yessin is a world-renowned pianist. He played more than three dozen times with the Boston Symphony Pops Orchestra under Arthur Fiedler, was a soloist with the New York Philharmonic, and played piano on numerous occasions as part of various television programs. In addition, he was the founding chair of the music department at the University of North Florida and professor of music until his retirement in 1998. In addition to all this, he is no stranger to volunteering. When he volunteered at Baptist Beaches Hospital in Jacksonville Beach, Florida, his initial job was to change the emergency room bed sheets. From sheet music to bed sheets. Quite a leap. He began to wonder if the Hospital could use his musical talents. It could. So, with a volunteer coordinator by his side, he'd ask patients if they wanted to hear a little piano music. If they said "Yes," Dr. Yessin trotted out a miniature electric keyboard and played either soothing pieces or energetic, lively ones, according to the patient's wishes.

Sometimes he'd play one of the two famous "Ave Marias" by Bach or Schubert, quiet, gentle pieces, or the "Turkish March" by Mozart, an energetic piece to lift the spirits. He says, "Many, many times, people would say, 'I feel so much better.' They would come to life!" He adds, "Often people would tell me, 'I used to play that!' or they'd remember that their parents played a particular piece. But most often, they said they forgot their pain for a while."

- You can help in a hospital setting without taking on duties that require a lot of walking or standing. Volunteer for clerical positions, assisting with mailings, filing, faxing, or compiling information. You can also be a friendly greeter at information desks, providing directions and creating a good first impression.

- Volunteering at least once a week is one of the greatest ways to achieve healing and wellness. Find something you are passionate about, set up a good schedule for yourself, and get into action. Libraries will embrace you; hospitals, senior centers, local theater groups, and humane societies will all be happy to have you sign on.

- If you enjoy books or newspapers, you might enjoy being a Radio Reader, reading live on the radio to the blind. Delivering Meals on

Wheels is gratifying, too. The possibilities are endless, and the rewards are, too.

- Volunteering with a member of the family can be a wonderful time to bond. An article in *Better Homes and Gardens*, November 2007,[37] had nifty ideas on volunteering your time with your kids. A few of these ideas include:
  - Visit the Binky Patrol (www.binkypatrol.org). You and a youngster could knit, quilt, crochet, or sew a blanket and then give it to a local Binky Patrol chapter or to a local hospital. The Patrol has great patterns on the Internet to choose from.
  - Another group, Warm Up America, collects knitted or crocheted sections and turns them into blankets. It's a great idea if doing an entire one is too much for you. Find out how to get involved with kids or on your own by visiting the website, www.warmupamerica.org. You'll find free, easy patterns and instructions. A senior center would be a wonderful venue for people to get together with others and knit for the homeless.
  - Becoming part of The Box Project (www.boxproject.org) lets you choose a family to whom you can send a box of food, clothing, and other items once a month. This is another wonderful way to instill the spirit of volunteerism into your kid or yourself. As the website says, it links families in need with families who care.
- *The Busy Family's Guide to Volunteering*, by Jenny Friedman, is a good place to start if you want to volunteer family style.[38]

Working at Work or Working at Home

I met Emma W. at a support group in the early 2000s. She came into the room in a wheelchair, pushed by her mother. It is rare when a person with peripheral neuropathy is unable to get around under her own steam, but Emma's hands and legs were pretty much nonfunctioning due to one of the more severe types of peripheral neuropathy. She had been a dental hygienist, but hadn't been able to work in a long time.

The majority of PNers can stay at their workplace, although for some it is not possible. Working out of the home may be the answer. For Emma, there was no choice. She says, "It took me a while to get used to not going into work. Illness can often be a family affair."

A strong case for staying at work if at all possible is made by Rosalind Joffe and Joan Friedlander in the book *Women, Work, and Autoimmune Disease*.[39] They say that if you are able to continue your work, try to do so. The camaraderie, the feelings of self-worth, the therapy that meaningful work provides—not to mention the paycheck—are all important reasons to think before you quit. These authors say that if you keep on working, you'll be in good company. The National Organization on Disability says 10 million Americans work despite a chronic condition.[40]

Yoga: A New Slant

For some with neuropathy, classic yoga positions aren't possible—too many problems with balance and flexibility. Believe it or not, there's something called "Laughter Yoga."

Not surprisingly, such classes started in India, when Dr. Madan Kataria, realizing the health benefits for both laughter and yoga, put them together. His student, Vishwa Prakash, went on to create a "laughter bank" of 100 exercises, such as "lion exercises," "hearty exercises," and "laughter for no reason." An article in the March 2008 edition of *Natural Awakenings–Northeast Florida*[41] says this type of yoga is all about mind and soul. The benefits to one's health reach both head and heart.

- Regulars at "yogalaff" classes feel a general wellness of being and are better able to manage the tensions and stress of daily life.

- Consider laughter yoga if your neuropathy makes you feel depressed.

Your Children: A Special Note to Parents

As I wind up this chapter, it occurs to me that this book focuses on older people and doesn't address children. We think of neuropathy as an adult person's ailment, but two of the human interest stories in Chapter 10 revolve around people whose memories go back to their childhood battles with peripheral neuropathy, and there must be thousands if not millions of similar voices out there.

A woman once drove 300 miles from Ft. Lauderdale to meet me at a Cracker Barrel in Jacksonville to discuss her child's neuropathy, which had started from birth. It's one thing to discover you have it after five or six decades of *not* having it, but to have it as a baby is heartbreaking for everyone involved.

Importantly, if your child has a hard time in sports and can't keep up with friends on a playing field, don't just listen to your pediatrician who says, "It's growing pains."

You can teach your children at an early age, perhaps around 6 or 7, that the more they focus on their pain—whether it's neuropathy or not—the worse the pain will seem and the more it will bother them. If you are anxious, your anxiety will transmit like lightning to your child. The book *Stop Being Your Symptoms*, by Doctors Bersky and Deans, may help you.[42] The information on hobbies and exercise found throughout this book, and some of the ideas from this chapter on wellness may also help you and your child cope more easily with neuropathy. See the For Further Reading section for even more inspiration.[43–45]

Zzzzz's Are All-Important

If diabetes runs in your family, keep in mind the importance of sleep. James Gangwisch, PhD, of Columbia University Medical Center, says even 1 hour less of sleep a night decreases insulin sensitivity, and that increases the risk of diabetes.[46] Seven to nine hours of sleep is the suggested amount.

One Final Word

Here's an anecdote about diabetes. A while back, Bev Anderson invited her podiatrist to a support group meeting. Thirty-three members showed up; a few of his patients were in the audience. In advance, Bev had told him that many in the group didn't have diabetes, but it didn't register.

When the meeting started, Bev asked, "How many of you have diabetes?" Three people raised their hands. The amazed doctor said, "What do I do now? I brought a presentation of the diabetic foot!" And the gracious Bev said, "Go right ahead with it. The three who are diabetic will especially benefit, and the rest of us will listen and learn, and appreciate that we don't have diabetes!" All of which is to say once again, neuropathy isn't all about diabetes. Not by a long shot.

For Further Reading

1. Dossey, Larry, MD. *The Extraordinary Healing Power of Ordinary Things: Fourteen Natural Steps to Health and Happiness*. New York: Harmony, 2006.

2. Simmons, Ronnie. "Exercise your mind." *Ideal Lifestyles*. Spring, 2008.

3. Gwinn, Eric. "Mind games." *The Chicago Tribune*, July 12, 2008.

4. Roberts-Grey, Gina. "Video games get smarter." *Arthritis Today*. March/April, 2008.

5. Davidson, Carolyn. *Word-a-Holic Quiz Book: Guess the Meaning of Real Words You Won't Believe*. West Conshohocken, PA: Infinity Publishing, 2005.

6. Roizen, Michael. F., and Mehmet C. Oz. *You: Staying Young: The Owner's Manual for Extending Your Warranty*. New York: Free Press, 2007.

7. Buffett, Warren. *Sunday Morning* (Television talk show). July 27, 2008.

8. Siegel, Bernie S. *Love, Medicine and Miracles: Lessons Learned About Self-Healing from a Surgeon's Experience with Exceptional Patients*. New York: Harper Perennial, 1990.

9. Cousins, Norman. *Anatomy of an Illness as Perceived by the Patient*. New York: W.W. Norton, 2001.

10. Rosenfeld, Arthur. *The Truth About Chronic Pain*. New York: Basic Books, 2003.

11. Carey, Benedict. "Learning how to reflect or not." *New York Times*. May 27, 2008.

12. Moyers, Bill. *Healing and the Mind*. New York: Doubleday, 1993.

13. Gorson, Kenneth. "Influenza vaccination in patients with neuropathy: Should you get a flu shot?" *Neuropathy News®*, September 2007.

14. Weiner, Eric. *The Geography of Bliss*. New York; Twelve/Hachette Book Group USA, 2008.

15. Tanner, Lindsey. "Who knew the bluebird of happiness was gray?" *The Florida Times-Union*. April 19, 2008.

16. McMahon, Darrin M. *Happiness: A History*. New York: Atlantic Monthly Press, 2005.

17. Martin, Paul, PhD. *The Healing Mind*. New York: Thomas Dunne/St. Martin's Press, 1997.

18. Groopman, Jerome, MD. *The Anatomy of Hope: How People Prevail in the Face of Illness*. New York: Random House, 2004.

19. LaRoche, Loretta. *The Joy of Stress*. DVD. Boston: WGBH, 2002.

20. Gilbert, Elizabeth. *Eat, Pray, Love*. New York: Viking, 2006.

21. Stein, Rob. "Midday naps to help fend off heart disease." *www.washingtonpost.com*. February 13, 2007.

22. Berman, Scott. "Depression, anxiety and fatigue in the neuropathy patient." *Neuropathy News®*, June 2002.

23. Cushing, Mims. *If You're Having a Crummy Day, Brush Off the Crumbs*. Kearney, NE: Morris Publishing, 2002.

24. Allan, Carrie. "Cat crisis." *All Animals*. Spring 2008.

25. *www.petsfortheelderly.org*. April 2008.

26. Benson, Herbert. *The Relaxation Response*. New York: HarperTorch, 1976.

27. "When happy becomes sad." *Better Homes and Gardens*, November 2007.

28. Kaplan, Francie. "Sing, sing a song ... sing out loud, sing out strong." *Arthritis Today*. March/April 2008.

29. Harrar, Sari. "Sing two songs and call me in the morning." *Oprah*, May 2008.

30. "Healing relationships." www.personaltransformation.com/Elkins.html. May 2008.

31. Scrimgeour, David. LAC "Into the calm." *Natural Solutions*, April 2008.

32. Harrington, Anne. *The Cure Within: A History of Mind-Body Medicine*. New York: W.W. Norton, 2008.

33. Pausch, Randy. *The Last Lecture.* New York: Hyperion, 2008.

34. Doughty, Rebecca. *Some Helpful Tips for a Better World and a Happier Life.* New York: Schwartz & Wade, 2008.

35. Orloff, Judith, MD. *Positive Energy: 10 Extraordinary Prescriptions for Transforming Fatigue, Stress, & Fear into Vibrance, Strength, & Love.* New York: Harmony Books, 2004.

36. Bailey, Simon T. *Release Your Brilliance.* New York: HarperCollins, 2008.

37. Odin, Anne. "Raise your hand." *Better Homes and Gardens.* November 2007.

38. Friedman, Jenny. *Busy Family's Guide to Volunteering.* New York: Robins Lane Press, 2003.

39. Joffe, Rosalind and Joan Friedlander. *Women, Work, and Autoimmune Disease.* New York: Demos Medical Publishing, 2008.

40. National Organization on Disability. www.nod.org.

41. Childs, Kim. "What's so funny about Yoga?" *Natural Awakenings-Northeast Florida.* March 2008.

42. Barsky, Arthur, MD, and Emily C. Deans, MD. *Stop Being Your Symptoms and Start Being Yourself: The 6-Week Mind-Body Program to Ease Your Chronic Symptoms.* New York: HarperCollins, 2006.

43. Kunz, Barbara and Kevin. *Complete Reflexology for Life.* London: DK Adult, 2007.

44. Remen, Rachel Naomi. *Kitchen Table Wisdom: Stories That Heal.* New York: Riverhead Books, 1996.

45. Remen Rachel Naomi. *My Grandfather's Blessings: Stories of Strength, Refuge, and Belonging.* New York: Riverhead Trade, 2001.

46. "Counting zzzzz's." *Good Housekeeping.* April 2008.

6

Hobbies: Escaping Symptoms through Distraction

Mims Cushing

The art of medicine consists of keeping the patient amused
while nature heals the disease.
—VOLTAIRE

When you were a child and had to stay home because of the flu, did you have fun reading comic books or movie magazines? Did you play cards with siblings? Practice a hobby you loved? It made sick time fly, didn't it? I hope you learned a lot about the importance of having hobbies to amuse yourself when you are not well. That is why this chapter—about diversions—is so important. Keeping yourself entertained with hobbies you love is an art.

Escaping Pain through Hobbies

Stephen Spielberg said, "Never lose your inner child." Hobbies—avocations—are the things we do because we want to, we love to. Wallace Stegner droned on through workdays in the insurance business, but he wrote poetry at night to give his life energy and purpose, and went on to became a renowned poet.

- During those times when you are having a bad neuropathy flare and don't feel like doing much, either you can do it anyway, and maybe that is the best thing to do, or you can get involved with something you love. Maybe you work during the day, so you must save your hobby as your after-supper evening treat. Let yourself retreat. And then re-treat yourself often. A weekend is also a wonderful time to become immersed in your hobbies.

- A hobby we become passionate about today is often something we loved when we were young. Figure out what appealed to you as a third grader and return to those moments of contentment. Give yourself permission to enjoy whatever gave you pleasure.

Your neuropathy may prevent you from doing certain things, but dig hard. Did you love to crayon? Try art if your hands are not affected. Did you adore your dog or cat? Adopt one for a while; save a pet's life and enhance your own. Maybe you liked to write poetry for the school literary magazine. Did you organize your life into collections of scrapbooks? Scrapbooking is very popular these days! Richard P., who has peripheral neuropathy, relishes spending hours creating 3- or 4-foot model ships. If you loved whittling as a child, try woodworking. Take a look at the following choices or think up your own:

Never Alone

Plenty of people don't have someone in their life who can play cards or games any old time of day or night. It's the lucky person who has developed the knack of enjoying her own company. These are often the ones who have found they've been given a gift: the gift of a hobby they love.

Art

- Many art books deal with therapy from a psychological viewpoint. Dabbling in paints is not going to help your feet from a physical standpoint, but if you paint, draw, or sculpt and it takes your mind off the pain, is there value in that? Yes. Is it quantifiable? No. Measurable? No. Will your neurologist take a tuning fork and find your nerves have more sensation? No. But if your hobby helps you escape your symptoms, none of that matters.

- More than books on theory, check out books on whatever medium appeals to you. Watercolor? Oil? Ceramics? Your community cultural center and senior center probably have classes you would enjoy. Jewelry making comes to mind, along with decoupage, tole painting, and so much more. If you're adventurous, think of crafts such as batik, beadwork, decorative tiling, painting on boxes or trays, or stenciling. Wander around the aisles of a nearby crafts store, and you'll be amazed at things to keep you busy if you need to be indoors because your neuropathy's being a pain.

- *The Complete Book of Home Crafts: Projects for Adventurous Beginners*, edited by Carine Tracanelli,[1] is a beautiful coffee table book that might inspire you to try something artistic. Well illustrated and presented in easy-to-follow steps, the book itself will decorate your table, even if you never get around to putting your own handiwork on your tabletop.

- Photography is another hobby that will provide you with hours of creativity. Don't just think of photography as taking pictures of the family. Take shots of the landscape, nature, birds, lakes, flowers, or animals. It can be a relaxing hobby. Put together a scrapbook. Use a theme: goofy shots of your pet, or photos of the changing-of-the-guard of birds around a lake.

Genealogy

My friend Sid walks, then rides his bike in the morning. In the afternoon, he happily sits at his computer working at his family tree. He has so much information about his ancestors, dating back to the 1600s, that he once put all the printouts on a wall in his house, until his wife said, "Enough already!"

Working on your "tree" can be an eye-opening adventure. Your family will love it and be intrigued, too. You can spend hours getting deeper and deeper into it. You may have so much fun doing detective work on past relatives that you ignore your existing ones. (Not a good plan.)

Here are some resources that can help you in your quest to know more about your ancestors:

- *Family Tree*, a bimonthly magazine, will provide you with dozens of tips and hours of enjoyment if you are a serious genealogist. To subscribe, visit www.familytreemagazine.com, or write to Family Tree, P.O. Box 421385, Palm Coast, FL 32142-7136. They will send you a free e-newsletter.

- For those people who have an international background, visit www.cyndislist.com to trace your worldwide roots.

- Trace your roots to Ellis Island through a visit to www.ellis island.org. The statistics from the New York Immigration port are open to you. More than 100 million U.S. citizens may trace their roots and look at images of ship documents that show what country an individual came from, in whose company he entered America, and who met him in New York.

- The U.S. Gen Web Project at www.usgenweb.com will give you links to the smallest historical societies in the smallest towns. You can research county marriage records and cemeteries.

- If you want to dig even deeper, visit www.findmypast.com, a U.K. resource that has a National Burial Index with records going back to 1538.

- To save the best for last, www.ancestry.com has five billion names! The site has everything from census records, certificates of birth and death, documents relating to immigration, and even pages from school yearbooks.

Writing about Your Illness

If the thought of writing makes your skin crawl, I understand. I dislike anything to do with math. If somebody told me I could cure my neuropathy by taking up higher mathematics, I'd say "Algebraic equations, be damned!" Then I'd crawl into my vacuum cleaner closet with a tub of Appletinis, settle down with my peripheral neuropathy, and hide in there. But if you find the idea of writing intriguing, give it a try.

Doing reflective writing about your illness has received serious consideration as excellent therapy for people suffering from trauma or chronic illness. Pat Stanley, who has an M.A. in Health Advocacy, works at the Program in Narrative Medicine at Columbia University in New York City (www.narrativemedicine.org). This program was established in 1996 by Rita Charon, and the core faculty consists of seven professionals. She says the patients' writing allows doctors, therapists, and families to absorb a person's inner feelings, emotions, and awareness. This is a tremendous help for professionals working to improve their patients' treatment. Narrative medicine workshops allow healthcare professionals from around the globe to train at the University and then bring the program back to their institutions. Pat Stanley is a avid believer in the power of putting your illness on paper. People feel better when they share their pain.

- Your writing might help your caretakers or close relatives better understand you. Consider sharing your work with them. It could be advantageous for everyone.

- "If you can talk you can write." Honestly. To make it easier, pretend you are writing to a friend. Not just a relative or any friend. Think big: write an essay or journal entry that Oprah, Barbara Walters, or Michelle Obama might read.

- If your hands are afflicted with neuropathy and writing with a pen or pencil is painful, try typing on a computer. You may be surprised to find that you can type on a keyboard with little or no pain.

If writing about your illness or essay writing isn't for you, simply write in a daily journal, particularly in a gratitude journal. A wonderful resource is *The Simple Abundance of Gratitude*, by Sarah Ban Breathnach.[2] She offers you five printed lines per day on which you write why the day made you feel better. The book offers you a list of "150 Often Overlooked Blessings" and includes things such as breakfast in bed, free samplings of wine at a local store, or perhaps a cozy day at home, listening to rain on the skylight. The granddaddy of all books on journaling is Ira Progroff's *At a Journal Workshop: The Basic Text and Guide for Using the Intensive Journal*. Never underestimate the value of journaling about your neuropathy.[3]

Does keeping a gratitude journal make a difference in your feelings of wellness? In *Thanks! How the New Science of Gratitude Can Make You Happier*, Robert Emmons,[4] a psychologist, used transplant patients to see if a gratitude journal helped their sense of well-being. Patients were told to record feelings. One group was also asked to write a list of five things every day that made them feel grateful and why.

After 21 days, people who had written about gratitude had a better sense of wellness. Emmons is quoted as saying: "Having a chronic medical condition puts one at risk for deteriorating mental health and a reduction in one's sense of general health and vitality is an indicator of this. Gratitude may serve as a buffer against these risks."[4]

- Don't make a 6-month commitment to write. Just write today.
- A gratitude journal doesn't have to be filled with lofty thoughts. The everyday flight of thought is what matters. Think up as few as three things to be grateful for, or as many as you like. Your entry might say "Today I am grateful for the cool breezes, for Lily's wagging tail that fans me, for Ray's e-mail funnygrams, for the rosemary oil I found at Fresh Market, and for the silly-looking anhingas drying their wings on Wendy's lawn."

Knitting and Other Needlework

If your hands constantly feel as though you are wearing gloves, of course knitting with small needles is out, but if you are housebound because of your feet, consider focusing your attention onto your hands by using large needles. Creating something as simple as a scarf or cap for a granddaughter, or making a hooked rug, can provide you with hours of pleasure. You can knit those chic, little knitted scarves in just a few hours using large needles, and you'll find them satisfying to create. Knitting is soothing.

Popular sites on knitting, needlework, and other handicrafts abound, and the materials to make interesting knitwear or crafts can be as close as your neighborhood store.

Music

Listening to music can calm you down or pick you up. Playing the piano or an instrument you played as a child is a great way to spend time, but your hands may not work as well as before. If your inner child has always wanted to play an instrument, try one. If you are musically gifted and have a good voice, join a choir or a music group.

The respected founder of The Center for Integrative Medicine, Andrew Weill, MD, recommends that you turn off the news once a week. He calls it a "news fast." Listen to music, buy flowers, read inspirational books, volunteer. These ideas come from a Harvard Medical School graduate, a renowned doctor, who believes that wellness results when you make time for art, keep in touch with nature, and take deep relaxing breaths. If you believe in alternative medicine, hunker down with one of his books.

So yes, when your neuropathy is annoying you, turn off the news on TV for a day and stop those yammering newscasters. Put on some music, and the atmosphere in your house will change. In *How to Talk With Your Doctor*, by Ronald Hoffman, MD,[5] he writes about the value of calming patients with music—pre-surgery, during surgery, and post-surgery. He says music reduces pain, lowers blood pressure and heart rate, and lessens anxiety and stress.

- If your neuropathy wakes you up and you are unable to relax at night, which is often the case, choose calming music, such as a soft classical piece. If you need livelier music to pick you up during the day, choose something like jazz or rock.

- It makes sense to listen to sounds you love, but once in a while experiment with change-of-pace music.

- Get your favorite CDs, divide them into categories—calming or lively—and keep them together in a special spot, so that you won't have to hunt for them.

- Hospice recommends that if you are feeling down or depressed, leave music on in your home most or all of the time. Sometimes too much silence can be deafening, unless you're meditating.

Reading

*I think, at a child's birth, if a mother could ask a fairy godmother to
endow it with the most useful gift, that gift would be curiosity.*
—ELEANOR ROOSEVELT

Emily Dickinson said, "There is no frigate like a book to take you miles away."
You can press the delete button on your neuropathy symptoms when you
become absorbed in a gripping mystery or romance or an amazing biography.
Bibliotherapy is a term coined by the famous psychiatrist Carl Menninger,
who suggested fiction and nonfiction would help patients cope with their ailments. As with music, sometimes we want funny, lively entertainment, while
at other times we want to be sent into deeper patterns of thought.

- If you love to read and especially love just-published books, I recommend the magazine *Bookmarks,* subtitled "For everyone who
  hasn't read everything."

- A free treat for readers is the catalog, *Bas Bleu.* If there's a book
  catalog that's more fun, I'd like to know about it. (*Bas bleu* in
  French means "blue stocking," a literary woman, and it's pronounced Bah Bluh.) The writing is witty and informal, and the
  books listed are special, not mainstream bestsellers. To get free
  monthly catalogs visit, www.basbleu.com, or call 800-433-1155.

- *Booklist: Recommended Reading for Every Mood, Moment and
  Reason* is the American Library Association's monthly scoop on
  what's good to read. It provides annotated lists to cater to everyone's tastes and personality. Google Booklist, and you can get a
  free online newsletter as well as one current magazine. The ALA
  calls itself an "irresistible book review site." I'll second that.

- If you're looking to sharpen your brain, *Book Smart: Your Essential
  Reading List for Becoming a Literary Genius in 365 Days*, by
  Jane Mallison, might be a great way to do just that.[6] You can order it
  through *Bas Bleu.* Read it to take a break from books on wellness.

- Ezra Pound calls a book "A ball of light in one's hand." You can collect an armful of light at your neighborhood Used Book Sales Days,
  organized by libraries and sometimes by college alumni groups as
  fundraisers.

Movies can provide *cinematherapy,* yet another approach to wellness.
While books and movies could just as easily be listed under the Wellness
chapter, reading and going to movies can be considered hobbies, as you can

collect them, figuratively or literally. Cinema lovers can read about this genre in *Reel Therapy, The Motion Picture Prescription: Rent Two Films and Let's Talk in the Morning,* by Dr. Gary Solomon.[7]

Dr. Solomon is a mental health therapist who invented the concept of cinematherapy. The books he has written do not address health issues, but rather emotional ones. Judging from the comments of many people with neuropathy, health issues often affect the emotions, which in turn affect relationships. In Dr. Solomon's books, he prescribes movies to help you deal with emotional issues. They are healing guides to help you resolve life's problems.

- If you believe laughter is the best therapy, then rent funny movies. Get yourself a video or DVD movie guide and flip through it to remind you of rib-tickling flicks to re-run. You can buy DVDs and videos (and music DVDs too) for $2 to $4 at some used book sales. (See more about laughter in Chapter 5.)

For Further Reading

1. Tracanelli, Carine. *The Complete Book of Home Crafts: Projects for Adventurous Beginners.* New York: New Burlington Books, 2000.

2. Ban Breathnach, Sarah. *The Simple Abundance Journal of Gratitude.* New York: Warner Books, 1996.

3. Progoff, Ira. *At a Journal Workshop: The Basic Text and Guide for Using the Intensive Journal.* New York: Dialogue House Library, 1975.

4. Emmons, Robert. *Thanks! How the New Science of Gratitude Can Make You Happier.* New York: Houghton Mifflin, 2007.

5. Hoffman, Donald L., MD. *How to Talk With Your Doctor.* Laguna Beach, CA: Basic Health Publications, 2006.

6. Mallison, Jane. *Book Smart: Your Essential Reading List for Becoming a Literary Genius in 365 Days.* New York: McGraw-Hill, 2007.

7. Solomon, Gary. *Reel Therapy, The Motion Picture Prescription: Rent Two Films and Let's Talk in the Morning.* Tampa, FL: Lebhar-Friedman, 2001.

7

Travel: Pack and Go Forth!

Mims Cushing

The world's a book and those who do not travel, read only one page.
—St. Augustine of Hippo

L t. Col. Eugene B. Richardson, USA Retired, calls himself a "flake" because every winter he longs for snow, even though he lives in Lake Placid, Florida. One January, despite his severe peripheral neuropathy (he has chronic inflammatory demyelinating polyneuropathy [CIDP]), he traveled with his wife and grandkids to hunt for the white stuff in the mountains of North Carolina. The mountainside is his secret place of peace and where he goes to daydream or meditate. The snow hid until the last day; nevertheless he and his family made memories every single hour. Gene learns something from every event in his life, and on this trip he learned that in cold weather—not extreme cold, which is damaging—he could walk more because the cold calms the muscles, reducing the inflammation. Yes, the 6-day trip was exhausting, but the exhilaration far outweighed any discomfort or fatigue.

Planning Ahead

- If your peripheral neuropathy is one of the more complicated varieties, you will have to plan ahead more than the person with a milder peripheral neuropathy problem who flings a toothbrush and a bathing suit into a carry-on and goes off to Aruba.

- If you have a medical problem in a foreign country, or even in the United States, it is essential that you have a tour director who can act knowledgeably and get help fast. Do your homework on this and hook up with a reliable tour.

- If you are going abroad, learn the language. The Mayo Clinic wrote in a newsletter about the value of travel for people with chronic illness and especially notes the value to your brain of learning a foreign language.

Plane Travel

Here are a few tips to get this chapter rolling: And by the way, remember to build lots of extra time into your plans, no matter how you travel.

- PNers should be vigilant about doing leg and foot stretches on long flights. Do not cross your legs, as that can decrease circulation. Ask for an aisle seat, so that you don't have to climb over your seat mate and take as many strolls as you dare.
- Travel with ample medication in your carry-on. You could be stranded and separated from your stowed luggage for a long time. And luggage has been known to get lost.
- Take along written prescriptions of all your meds, an extra pair of glasses, and your latest eyeglass prescription.
- Bring anything you need to lubricate your eyes, as the atmosphere in the plane's cabin can be a problem. This especially applies to those who have the neuropathic eye issue called *Sjögren's syndrome*, which causes irritatingly dry eyes and mouth because of an inflammation of the salivary ducts and numerous other problems.
- Some airlines using commuter planes make you climb down the airport's stairs at the terminal and take a bus to their little plane (such as Delta's ComAir at LaGuardia). You do *not* have to use the stairs. Ask airport personnel, and eventually someone will escort you to the terminal's elevator. It's not just for people in wheelchairs. Lugging a carry-on down steep stairs when your balance is off can be downright dangerous.

Trains

If you're interested in rail travel, Amtrak has excellent information for every type of trip you can think of. And check out Candy Harrington's trio of books, listed at http://www.demosmedpub.com/results.aspx?srch=candy%20&titl=1&desc=1&auth=1&isbn=1.

Cruises

If you're a bit wobbly on foot and leery about traveling on a moving ship, take solace in the words from *The Unofficial Guide to Cruises*,[1] in which authors

Showker and Sehlinger say that, if you can walk about in a hotel, you can probably walk on a cruise ship without problems.

Crutches, however, can be dicey in a rolling sea. A walker is better; a collapsible wheelchair perhaps the best. The huge mega-ships have wide open spaces on board and plenty of passageway space. Some of the smaller luxury ships should be fine, too. Think twice about taking a barge cruise if you have trouble getting around. No matter what cruise you take, ask the cruise line about matters of your safety before you leave. While most ships today have excellent facilities in their on-board hospitals, small ships, such as freighters that carry fewer than 12 passengers, come with limited medical treatment, say Showker and Sehlinger.

Some cabins have showers with chairs or stools, and some tubs have devices you can grip for getting and out with ease. Luxury staterooms can have very deep tubs that might cause you a problem, so ask your travel agent.

- Be sure to request a cabin near the elevator. As a PNer, you'll be glad you did.

- Taking out travel health insurance is a good idea.

- Always carry extra medications.

Getting a Handicapped Placard: Still on the Road . . .

- Do you need a handicapped placard to hang on your rear view mirror? Here's a test: If your discomfort is so great that you'd rather stay at home than have to walk with pain from a parking lot to stores, movies, or events, then yes, you need one . . . on that one specific day. That doesn't mean you must use it every day. A doctor told PNers in the *Neuropathy News* to get one if it's necessary, and then use it only when you must.

- You need your doctor's consent first; then get the placard at the Motor Vehicle Bureau for a nominal fee. Please do not loan your placard to anyone. You are doing a disservice to all who really need a handicapped space. Try to shop when parking lots are less crowded.

- Bring your handicapped placard with you when you travel, and don't leave it in a rental car. In some states, your hanging placard might not be accepted, so bring along a doctor's note in case you must go to the DMV.

- Do not drive with the placard hanging on the mirror. You can be ticketed for that.

Free Wheeling

On the *Today* show, March 26, 2008, a spokesperson said the Wheelchair Foundation had recently given wheelchairs to 100,000 people in the United States. In all, the top-notch charity has delivered 710,229 wheelchairs between 2000 and 2007. It is estimated that 100 million children and adults need them. People who donate $150 to the Foundation, which has a four-star rating are, in effect, giving a wheelchair to a needy person here or abroad. The goal is to deliver one million in all by 2012.

Visit wheelchairfoundation.org or write Wheelchair Foundation, 3820 Blackhawk Road, Danville, CA 94506-4617, if you or someone you know needs the freedom and mobility that a wheelchair provides. Or call the organization at 925-791-2340.

This 'n' That

- Zip-It Gear, of San Diego, California, sells traveler's socks that have a zipper-closed security pocket on one sock, where you can stash credit cards and money. It won't set off metal detectors in airports and is great for those who don't want a heavy handbag or tote that will be difficult on the hands. The socks are crew height, have an impact-absorbing sole, and wick moisture away. They are 80% poly-olefin, 15% nylon, and 5% spandex. You can also buy waist belts or neck belts that hold money and ID. Visit the company's site at www.zipitgear.com.

- If you want to take only a credit card, a few bills, and a key as you walk about, sneak your stuff into the heel of specially designed sandals. The organization that sells them is Reef for Project Blue, which helps protect our coastlines worldwide.

- Visit City Sports at www.citysports.com to browse a huge inventory of shoes, sports bras, and much more that can make traveling easier, more comfortable, and more enjoyable.

- Sun-protective clothing is a hot item. If you're out in the sun every day, it can get old to have to rub on creams and lotions all the time. Coolibar brand clothing blocks many harmful UVA rays and is recommended by the Skin Cancer Foundation. Go to www.coolibar.com. They have wonderful hats for every occasion, and plenty of shirts and slacks for men and women.

How's Your Driving?

A PNer I'll call Debbie plowed her car into the car in front of hers, which in turn plowed into the car in front of him at a red light because she didn't realize she hadn't put enough pressure (a neuropathy issue) on the brakes. No one was hurt, but her car's front end had to be overhauled.

- If you feel a bit uncoordinated when you drive, or if your ankles, feet, or legs are experiencing weakness, or if you have a loss of sensation, you do not have to give up driving. A driver rehabilitation specialist may be available in your area. Contact the Association for Driver Rehabilitation Specialists (ADRS) at 877-833-0427 or visit www.nmeda.org/consumers/htm, the National Mobility Equipment Dealer's Association.

- A driver rehabilitation specialist can evaluate whether or not you need hand controls and will train you how to use them. You can discuss the right vehicle for your wheelchair or scooter. You want to be independent, and advice from ADRS might make this possible.[2]

If Debbie's Story Isn't Bad Enough, Here's Mine

One day, after a few months of being on pain medication that made me very sleepy, I was driving home. I was only 10 minutes away. I had fought sleep all the way. It's a terrible way to drive, closing one eye to catnap, then closing the other, but I just wanted to get home. On A1A, in a blinding rain storm, I stopped at a red light, and thought, *I'll just close my eyes until the light changes.*

Suddenly, I heard pounding on my window. I rolled it down a crack, and a man hollered above the rain, "Are you all right? I saw you didn't drive on when the light turned green, and I came around to see if you're OK." I had fallen asleep when the light was red and stayed asleep when it turned green. You can be sure I never drive when I am in the least bit sleepy any more.

- The National Sleep Foundation's Sleep in America study reported that 32% of Americans "drive drowsy."[3] Be aware of what drivers around you are doing and not doing.

- Flexibility from your neck to your feet is tremendously important when you drive. A recent study by the Yale University School of Medicine showed when people exercise every day, they make 37% fewer critical driving errors.[3] For 3 months, approximately 170 adults aged 70 and older who drive once a week or more had their reflexes tested as they drove in various settings. During that time, they exercised to gain flexibility. The results showed exercise helps older drivers maintain or improve their driving skills.

- The American Association of Retired People (AARP) offers driver-safety courses at sites around the nation for adults older 50. The

American Automotive Association (AAA) has an online self-rating test designed to be taken by drivers 55 and older. Auto insurance companies give you a rate reduction for taking these driver safety courses.

- The Centers for Disease Control (CDC) says senior drivers should perform a minimum of 30 minutes of aerobic exercise at least four times a week to offset deteriorating changes in cognitive ability.[3]

Elderhostel

Elderhostel is a not-for-profit travel organization committed to building knowledge and widening horizons for adults 55 and older. It can also be of vital assistance to a PNer with needs for special equipment. You can call the main number to find out what options are available and where at 877-426-8056.

- Elderhostel, which features "Adventures in Lifelong Learning" at a "remarkable price" can tell you what places offer grab bars in baths or special seats in showers. They will accommodate your dietary needs, and perhaps make it possible for you to travel.

- The listings in Elderhostel's huge catalog note what accommodations are "handicapped-friendly," what tours involve considerable walking, and how long the average walks might take. It also indicates if walks are on uneven terrain and not appropriate for a wheelchair. Call toll-free at 877-426-8056 or enroll online at www.elderhostel.org.

Resources for Travelers

- The International Association for Medical Assistance (IAMA) can supply you with a list of English-speaking doctors in foreign countries; call 716-754-4883. This organization can also tell you where they have been trained: in the United States, Great Britain, or Canada. Take along the name of your doctor and phone number in case you have a medical issue and the doctors need to confer. The Association provides other helpful information, such as whether the drinking water is safe, if there is a malaria risk, and if you need immunization.

- Travelin' Talk Network (931-552-6670), for a nominal fee, will send you a quarterly newsletter that includes numerous travel tips for people with special issues. Write to founder Rick Crowder at P.O. Box 3534, Clarksville, TN 37043-3534, to become a member and discover how people can help one another if a traveler needs help on a trip.

- Adventurers should check out Wilderness Inquiry at 800-728-0719. Located in Minnesota, it sponsors wilderness trips for people with chronic physical problems. Visit their website at www.wildderness-inquiry.org for more information.

- A more generic aid is *Directory of Travel Agencies for the Disabled*, written by Helen Hecker.[4] It lists travel agents who are specialists in arranging vacations for those with health issues. The agents do not arrange one-size-fits-all trips, and will listen to your needs. To obtain a copy of the directory, write to Twin Peaks Press, P.O. Box 129, Vancouver, WA 98666-0129.

Eugene Richardson's Eight Tips on Travel

Richardson says take your neuropathy along and Travel, with a capital T. Keep going and don't give up. His advice:

- If you overly worry about your neuropathy on a trip, you could miss some of life's miracles.

- The best humor is often found in the common, simple events of traveling, providing moments for a good laugh or two—at life, at yourself.

- Never take your illness so seriously that it overwhelms you. You are much more than your illness or disabilities. Travel can help divert you.

- Thinking of the worst that can happen tomorrow is a sure-fire way to throw yourself into a state of helplessness and ruin a vacation.

- Don't be driven by the fear of what might be around the bend by saying, "Tomorrow will be worse. I just know it." That helps nothing, at home or away.

- Travel has a way of helping us discover what we need to know.

- Travel gives rise to surprises that we could miss if we sit at home wallowing in despair, anger, and negativity.

- Hope is always a possibility. Besides, there is today, and if there is today, there is hope. Keep traveling!

For Further Reading

1. Showker, Kay, with Bob Sehlinger. *The Unofficial Guide to Cruises: Lines & Ships Ranked & Rated, Best Cruise Deals*. New York: John Wiley & Sons, 2007.

2. Meyers, Mary Beth. "When neuropathy affects driving." *Neuropathy News*®, January 2008, page 14.

3. Sirianni, Ann. Living Smart: "How Exercise Can Keep You 'Fit to Drive.'" *Green Valley News and Sun*, 42, March 29, 2009.

4. Hecker, Helen. *Directory of Travel Agencies for the Disabled*. Vancouver, WA: Twin Peaks Press, 1991.

8

Caretakers:
Helping You to Help Others

Mims Cushing

What do we live for if it is not to make life
less difficult for each other.
—GEORGE ELIOT

In his memoir about living with multiple sclerosis, *Blindsided: Lifting a Life Above Illness, A Reluctant Memoir,* Richard M. Cohen[1] says illness is a family affair. A family that denies a chronic illness will eventually have to grapple with bigger issues—anger, resentment, depression. The sooner family members climb on board the Chronic Illness train, the better off everyone will be. Cohen says coping is an art. Perhaps it is also a science.

In more critical cases of peripheral neuropathy, if family cannot help, a caretaker is needed, although the percentage of PNers needing home health care is small. At a support group meeting, sometimes I see a gentle and loving look in the wife's or husband's eyes and think how blessed are they. You're lucky if you can be cared for by a loved one, treated with compassion by the one who knows you best. Not everyone is so fortunate. That's where professional caretakers come into the picture. And some of them become best friends with the person needing care. Other combinations don't work out. Floyd M. was one of the lucky ones.

When Floyd took a stress test, he was stunned to learn that he wouldn't be leaving the hospital that day. He needed a triple bypass. He sailed through the surgery, went home after a while, and was cared for by a nurse who changed his bandages for about a week or so.

Caretaking from the Patient's Point of View

Floyd, who just turned 80, says, "After the nurse left, I had to rely on a person from the church, a shepherd, around the clock, whom I wore out before I could get someone from a home health care agency. And then Esther came into my life. It was wonderful." One of the things Esther did was clean his house. He says, "My house was so clean I couldn't stand it!"

When I talked to Floyd, 3 weeks after his bypass, he said it took time to adjust to Esther. "We worked out a system. I hid in my computer room while she cleaned up. She'd tease me that she wanted to lock me in a room while she worked." Floyd says women are amazing, coming in and taking charge and getting things done. After some time, Esther came in once a month or so for a couple of months. Floyd says, "I am independent and driving again, but I'll look forward to seeing Esther here and there."

- Floyd's caveat is, "You have to kind of get dressed decently when you have someone coming to care for you. If you respect her, she will respect you."

- Prepare for a period of adjustment while you and your caretaker(s) work things out.

Caretaking from the Caretaker's Point of View

Leeann W., 68, has been a caretaker for more than 20 years. She took care of her parents' friends, all of whom lived in Massachusetts. Now, dividing her time between the northeast and southeast, she continues to care for people. Of all those she's cared for, she is most fond of RosaLee, who was in her 90s when Leeann began working for her.

RosaLee had neuropathy that affected her feet and legs, but not her hands. Leeann says, "When I cared for her, she always, no matter what her pain level was, walked from her apartment at a retirement facility to the dining room. No cane. No walker."

RosaLee's neuropathy caused numbness, which affected her balance, and she was in a good deal of discomfort, but she never complained. She was constantly on the go. Leeann says, "She was always organizing things. She worked on the facility's newsletter and rallied a group of people in a sewing group to put quilts together that would go to the Wellness Center for the very ill."

When the two of them went to KMart to get materials for the quilts, RosaLee would buy an armload of stuffed animals for the severely ill. "They loved her. When RosaLee was 95, she and I went on a cruise that left from Savannah. By then, she was on a walker. It was a sight to see her getting around on those cobblestones."

Leeann says RosaLee spoiled her. She would love to work for another RosaLee because she was so generous in spirit and uncomplaining, never negative about anything. "She never dwelled on her neuropathy, and managed to keep busy right up until the very end." RosaLee died at the age of 97.

- Leeann says, "The most important quality a caretaker should have is that she must be a good listener. The second quality is patience."
- "You Talk. I Will Listen." That's a perfect mantra for a caretaker. Or anyone.

If You Are Being Cared For in Your Home

No matter who cares for you, you need to do a self-check. Ask yourself:

- Are you letting your caretakers get some down time?
- If relatives in your home have a full-time job and care for you on weekends and evenings, it can be exhausting. Give them some slack. Don't wear them out.
- Do you take them for granted? Caregiving can be overwhelming, sometimes exasperating. A word of appreciation goes a long way.
- Do you understand their limitations? You need to know what they can and cannot do.
- Do you have backups in case they cannot care for you?
- Remember: Be Kind. Let Your Caretaker Unwind (apologies to Blockbuster).

If You Are a Caretaker

- Become as informed as you can about neuropathy. Discover what it's all about.
- It is essential that you take care of yourself. Eat right, and keep your sense of well-being intact. Indulge yourself periodically with a movie or night out with friends. Keep the balance in your life that worked for you before you started caretaking.
- Sleep is all-important. Take daytime naps when you must be up at night.
- Exercise will refresh you and keep you going. If there's a dog in the household, walk it around the block a couple of times.
- Don't let your diet or your belly go to pot. If you are doing the cooking, make healthful foods you both can enjoy.

- Don't ignore your own health. Maintain your own schedule of visits with doctors.

- Don't sweat the small stuff. Perfectionism will drag you and the whole household down.

Dianna Turker, former Jacksonville director of marketing for ComForcare Senior Services, a nationwide company, knows first-hand what it is like to care for a patient at home. Her mother-in-law came from Turkey to the United States for 6 months to greet Dianna's baby. Within a short time, the new grand-mother had a brainstem stroke that paralyzed her left side. The woman could barely talk, and she only spoke Turkish.

Dianna, with her husband's help, cared for her mother-in-law around the clock in the hospital, and then for 8 years at home. Turker says, "She never lost her temper or her sense of humor. She trusted and respected me, and I don't regret a minute of that time with her." Dianna's tips can serve any care-taker well:

- "Be sure you go to a health care agency that is licensed, insured, and bonded.

- "If you want to age in your own home and want a caretaker, go to an agency that insists on getting personal references from all employees. It should do background checks and drug testing, not just screening. Screening means the applicant is asked if they do drugs, whereas testing involves a urine sample.

- "You don't have to take the first person the agency sends. If there's any conflict or you're not happy, talk to a supervisor. Patients' desires must come first.

- "See that your caretaker keeps a balance in her life, so that she doesn't burn out. Caretakers must be able to care for themselves, as well as you."

Attention Must Be Paid to Caretakers

According to the National Family Caregivers Association, more than 50 mil-lion people serve as caregivers to chronically ill and the elderly. The National Alliance for Caregiving and the American Association of Retired People (AARP) say 44 million of those working as caretakers are unpaid. Paid or unpaid, caregivers need attention.

The caretaking role can be challenging and difficult. If there is a care-taker in your home, give her a respite. Make sure she understands she does-n't have to respond to every need. The local Council on Aging might be able to help by sponsoring support group meetings for caregivers. Encourage friends or relatives to enter the picture, so that your caretaker can let go of some responsibilities.

Here are tips a family member might employ to relieve other family members who are assuming the major effort of caretaking:

- Offer them a break. Say, "There must be something I can do for you. What will you let me do?" Don't just say, "Let me know if there's anything I can do."

- Can you bring lunch or dinner? Or, even better, set up a group of meal providers and a schedule.

- Suggest doing a load of laundry or ironing.

- Pick up groceries, take clothes to a dry cleaner, restock pet supplies, go to the post office.

- Bring or send a care package. For a woman, fill it with nurturing things: potpourri, hand lotion, bath gel, fleece socklets, a special magazine, air freshener, a packet of nuts or mints or a chocolate bar, a mini bottle of wine, a paperback. Or, bring over a little bouquet of flowers. For a man, well, you have to be a little more creative. Find out what his interests are. If he likes cars, give him auto maintenance products, or magazines about fitness or cars or boating. Food always works.

Help Yourself, Help Others

It's been shown that helping others makes you feel good and even boosts your immune system.
- The Web site for paid caretakers is the National Family Caregivers Association at www.nfcacares.org.

Visitor Etiquette

To share often and much ... to know even one life has breathed easier because you have lived. This is to have succeeded.
—Ralph Waldo Emerson

If you want to pop over and visit someone who can't do much because of her neuropathy, go the extra mile and do a few chores as well. Ask if you can empty the dishwasher, or maybe stack it and run it, fold clean clothes, change the bed linens, empty garbage pails, bring big pails out to the curb on garbage day. Can you mow? Rake? Shovel? Change a litter box? Time is a gift.

You could give your visitee a coupon book with chores you can do. The patient calls when she needs a special chore to be done. And one last thing: When you visit, less is better. If your visit is too long, you can wear people out. Leave with them wanting more.

Saying the Right Thing

On the cover of Susan P. Halpern's book *The Etiquette of Illness*,[2] Bill Moyers writes, "This is the most helpful book for hard times that I have read in years." The book's subtitle is "What to Say When You Can't Find the Words." Sometimes your closest family members just don't understand. Maybe you've been in remission, but the tough days are back. Maybe they are wondering why you aren't your old self any more because you can't play tennis, do chores the way you used to, or . . . fill in the blank.

Need help? Find some help in framing what you want to say from the tips listed in the accompanying box.

Speak Up

Eight Things You Can Tell Your Family and Friends

- I hear how worried you are.
- I hear how distressed you are with my slow recovery.
- There is no time limit on my recovery.
- I am sorry I can't respond to that.
- That is not a question you can ask.
- I find that hurtful.
- I'll let you know when I know.
- What are you trying to say to me?

What You Can Tell Your Ailing Friend

- I am here with you through this.
- It's OK to cry.
- Take time with your sadness.
- You don't have to be cheerful all the time.
- I love you.

Quoted with permission from *The Etiquette of Illness*, by Susan Halpern, Bloomsbury, 2004.

Something as simple as a quiet touch of your hand on a person's shoulder can mean so much. It can almost have a healing quality.

Belle C. has a phrase she uses for people needing encouragement. She says, "I am cheerleading for you." Sometimes a cheerleader is the best thing a caretaker can be.

For Further Reading

1. Cohen, Richard M. *Blindsided: Lifting a Life Above Illness A Reluctant Memoir.* New York: HarperCollins, 2004.

2. Halpern, Susan P. *The Etiquette of Illness: What to Say When You Can't Find the Words.* New York: Bloomsbury, USA, 2004.

9

The Neuropathy Association's Self-help Groups

Mims Cushing

Together, we can beat this disease.
—ONE OF THE NEUROPATHY ASSOCIATION'S MOTTOS

Visiting a Meeting: What Goes On?

It is 10 o'clock on the second Saturday of the month, March 8, 2008. As I drive along, I'm glad the torrential rains have stopped and we face only strong winds, which help dry up impromptu ponds decorating the banks of the roads. I'm headed toward the Neuropathy Association's Jacksonville support group, which meets 11 months a year. One man, Ken Davis, has come to meetings for nine years. He lives in Gainesville. The trip takes him 4 hours.

I began that support group in 1999. With dozens of cities around the United States having these Neuropathy Association support groups, I felt that Jacksonville, Florida, a city of almost a million residents, needed one, if not a dozen. I'd just been diagnosed with neuropathy, and I wanted to talk to others who had it, too. Irene Beer, a volunteer at The Neuropathy Association's headquarters, sent me a flood of information on how to start a support group, and she addressed my numerous concerns. She, too, has peripheral neuropathy. Irene told me to write publicity for local newspapers, which I did. I told readers we would meet at what was then known as the Mayo Clinic's St. Luke Hospital in Jacksonville.

At the first meeting, six of us showed up, none of whom had any idea what to expect, especially me. We did know we were in the same boat: We all had neuropathy. No, that's not true. As we went around the table to identify ourselves, we came to the last woman, who sheepishly said, "I don't have neuropathy. I am in the hospital visiting my husband who just had heart surgery. I decided to walk about a little bit. I saw your door was open, and noticed the coffee and doughnuts. I thought I'd just see what the meeting was about." She said she'd never heard about peripheral neuropathy. So, along with the rest of us, she settled in. We were happy that one more person on the planet would learn about peripheral neuropathy.

The meeting began. Being a word person, I was conscious that most of the attendees pronounced "peripheral" as "purr-I (short i)-fee-al," which told me this disease didn't have a lot of press.

What's In a Name?

You need to pronounce your ailment accurately! It's *per-i-fur-al*, accent on the short "i." Although some have said it should be called "perpetual" neuropathy!

After a few meetings, we realized that we wanted someone to answer medical questions. Sympathizing, empathizing wasn't enough. We were seeking answers. Neurologist Alan Berger, MD, agreed to sit in at one meeting. (Emphasis on "*one.*") Call him The Man Who Came to the Support Group. To this day, almost every month, he stays for an extra hour and a half to answer questions. He is also now director of a Neuropathy Association-designated center. In addition, Karen Perrin, outreach coordinator for Parkinson's disease and neuropathy, reminds members via e-mail of upcoming meetings.

I knew one thing for sure: People should not, must not, leave the meeting feeling down. Some people who have attended self-help meetings for other issues tell me, "It was such a downer. I never went back."

I understand some neurologists tell their patients not to go meetings because it could make them depressed. That is infuriating! These doctors have never been to a meeting, yet they condemn it?

In the fall of 2005, I stepped down after leading the group for 6 years. My feeling is that new blood should take the reins of any group after a period of time. My own neuropathy had calmed down so much I couldn't relate as well to the newcomers. I didn't realize then that peripheral neuropathy can buzz off for a while and then reappear as often as it feels like it.

Today's meeting has 15 people in attendance. Some groups across the United States have many more attendees, but the numbers aren't as important as how much knowledge people get from each meeting. Some PNers take the information they seek and leave after attending a few times, feeling they have learned enough. They come wanting cures and definitive answers, but absolutes are not part of this disease. Support groups ... support.

On this Saturday, Dr. Michael Pulley, assistant professor, Department of Neurology, and director of the Electromyogram (EMG) Laboratory at the University of Florida, is standing in for Dr. Berger.

Getting Underway

The support group members mill about for a few minutes, pouring coffee, getting snacks, and then taking a seat in a semicircle. Dr. Pulley answers questions. I've included a small sample of the Qs and As, here, since they're probably the most commonly asked:

Suzanne: How do you know when to stop doing tests?

Dr. Pulley: That's a good question. I try to leave it up to the patient. Some people have to have all the tests in the book. They really want to get to the bottom of things, and will even request a biopsy, which is taken from the side of the foot. There is one good reason to do a biopsy, and that is to check for vasculitis, an inflammation in the blood vessels, which can cause a stroke in your nerve. The third of the people who have vasculitis may present like all the others.

The main thing is that, if there are no clues in the blood work, if it's all negative and there's no pain, then it's pointless to do a biopsy. It is important for patients to continue to have basic cancer screenings such as mammograms, colon cancer tests, pap smears, and chest X-rays. Occasionally, neuropathy is a sign of cancer.

A glucose tolerance test (GTT) is a good idea if there's diabetes in the family and the GTT lets us see how the body handles sugar. Neuropathy is extremely common in people who have diabetes.

Dick: Does diet have an effect on neuropathy?

Dr. Pulley: It is almost impossible to prove if diets affect neuropathy. Studies are being done now.

Margaret: I certainly feel better when I eat less sugar.

Paul, interrupting (Paul is Margaret's husband): Well, Margaret eats every carbohydrate in the book. I mean, she will pass up a steak in order to eat carbos!

Dr. Pulley: I would absolutely say cut out sugar if you have fewer symptoms, but as I said, studies on the effects of diet are going on now.

Emily: I have a concern. I have drop foot. Where does this go? I've done all the studies. Can you slow this? Where is this leading? Are there treatments to slow the progression?

Dr. Pulley: Braces passively raise your foot. An AFO—ankle foot orthosis—is a plastic device you put in the front or the back of your leg. It can be a nuisance to some, but it helps others. It's about 50/50. One of the simplest is the Dorsi-Strap, and it's pretty ingenious. It's basically a lot of Velcro wrapped around the lower leg. A long string is put through the laces of the shoe and attaches to the Velcro. It helps the patient move the toes up and down.

Ed: I have a lot of pain. What about using a morphine pump for chronic pain?

Dr. Pulley: The goal with the pump is to put less of the drug in your system. It gives you a constant level of the drug. The concentration goes directly into your spine, not into your brain.

After the Q&A session, Dr. Pulley discusses the wild variables with neuropathy: at one end of the spectrum, it never bothers people; it never changes their lifestyle. At the other end, it forces them into completely overhauling how they live their life.

The questions continue, with someone bringing up the fact that neuropathy worsens at night, interfering with a person's sleep. You lie down to rest and you really notice the burning and pain. Or, you sit down to relax and the symptoms appear. Dr. Pulley explains that your brain doesn't have to think so hard when you are resting, so it focuses on your feet. Someone comments that it's like when a woman is pregnant and rushing around all day. She wonders why the baby kicks more at night. Maybe it doesn't; she just notices it more.

It's 11:30 A.M., and the doctor winds up by telling us to modify the way we do things. We have heard these tips many times before, but it cannot be repeated enough:

- Control your alcohol intake. Too much damages the nerves.
- Watch your sugar intake.
- Be cautious stepping on and off curbs. Always pick up your feet.
- Some neuropathies are treatable, which is why a doctor's evaluation is essential.

Just before we stand to leave, he calls out to the woman with drop foot. He's noticed her crossed legs and gently chides, "Don't cross your legs! It's not good for you." Further thoughts from Dr. Pulley:

- It's essential to stretch the Achilles tendon. Maintain your range of motion.

- Point your toes up and down several times a day, otherwise your foot might end up pointing downward.

- Take a towel, put it around your instep, and pull up on it.

Think about this comment an attendee made, if you're considering attending a group meeting: "These meetings are great. How many people can have a cup of coffee with their doctor on a Saturday morning and ask them whatever they want?"

Could You Be a Group Leader?

Absolutely. You can be as energetic and as involved a leader as you want to be. It helps if people have said you are enthusiastic, easy-going, embracing, and supportive. It's not hard to lead if you have the desire to help. You need to care, and the rest is easy. Many "chores" can be delegated. Here are a few tips:

- The first thing you need is The Neuropathy Association Support Group Leaders Manual. This 18-page booklet will answer all your questions. Contact the Association at supportgroups@neuropa-thyy.org for help with getting your group started and becoming part of their national network.

- Choose a central location such as a church, office, school, bank, or other easily accessible building.

- See if you can find a neurologist who will commit to monthly meetings, or find a team of doctors who will alternate. Plenty of groups thrive without having a monthly doctor visit. You may prefer to have speakers or a series of doctors in attendance from time to time.

- You cannot answer medical questions, but you or other members can be supportive about resources in the community and suggest recommendations for doctors.

- Do not let one person monopolize the conversation.

- Remind people nothing personal should leave the room. People must feel they are in a safe haven.

- Do not restrict members to people with peripheral neuropathy. Let family members or caretakers come, too.

- Get members involved. Ask what they want to get out of the meeting and for suggestions regarding speakers and topics.

- Collect $1 or $2 each time to go toward coffee and snacks. At year's end, if money is left over, consider donating it to The Neuropathy Association. If it's a small amount, buy get-well cards for ailing members.

- Hand out flyers and ask people to put them in doctors' offices with their permission. The Neuropathy Association will send you some. Call 212-692-0662 to request flyers and other literature.
- Ask for several volunteers. They can sign up to be:
  - Greeters to make new and returning members feel welcome
  - Refreshment organizers
  - "Telephoners" to call people who are sick
  - E-mailers to tell people about the next meeting
  - Public relations persons to tell newspapers about the meeting: date, time, place, and speaker. Know papers' deadlines; introduce yourself to calendar editors.

Leading Your First Support Group Meeting: Eight Things You Should Know

- Don't be dismayed if only a few people show up. "If you build it, they will come."
- Create a database. Everyone should sign in each time.
- Let people chat before the meeting starts.
- Introduce yourself when people are seated; say why you started the group.
- Go around the room and let the new people introduce themselves and talk about their peripheral neuropathy. No more than 5 minutes per person.
- End your meeting on an upbeat note. Very important: If it's been a difficult meeting, perhaps a depressing one, talk about a local event people can look forward to: a book sale, a pet expo, a fair, concert, or an antiques festival—anything so people won't leave dispirited. Keep a bunch of jokes with you for every meeting, and end with one once in a while. It takes practice to turn a meeting that's become a downer into an "upper."
- Type up a bulletin with tips you've picked up at the support meeting, or find someone who likes to write to send one or e-mail it. Perhaps tape the meeting for people who have missed it and give it to them the following month.
- Finally, embrace your group. Respect your members. And lead with grace, knowledge, and compassion.

- Pick a date and time that works for everyone. It should be in the evening or on Saturday mornings. One meeting a month, perhaps with a break in the summer, works well.

- Limit meetings to one or one-and-a-half hours.
- Bring a coffee pot, creamers, and sugar packets if they are not supplied. Some organizations do supply them—a real plus.
- Buy name badges in bulk and use them every time.
- Try to get the local newspaper to write a feature article, including photos of a meeting. Get attendees' permission.

A Post-Meeting Chat with "Don"

I am including this story about Don, but only after a considerable amount of thought. I think it is accurate to say Don's life with his peripheral neuropathy is out of control. I wrote these observations after talking to him one day after a meeting. Do you feel the way he does?

Don is living in chronic, demoralizing pain. Many people in such groups are in pain similar to Don's, but his is an extreme case. Don is 41. Three years ago, he loved extreme sports, jumping out of airplanes and wakeboarding.

Because of his neuropathy, he and his wife are barely functioning as a couple. He accuses her of being unfeeling; she accuses him of talking constantly about his pain. She doesn't want to hear about it any more. At one point, he made a concentrated effort to stop talking about it. Tears of frustration rolled down his cheeks as he walked around the house while she ignored him. He is unable to control his emotions. His wife often yells at him to complete a job, such as working on their mobile home. "What are you doing? Get off the couch," she says. Don literally can't continue because of the pain, despite medication. He has had to leave four or five jobs unfinished.

They went to a therapist and, after seven or eight sessions, with Don being told how negative he was, he quit. "It wasn't doing any good," he said. He was not giving recommended alternatives, such as acupuncture or biofeedback, a chance.

Don and his wife are leaving on a trip soon. Don is not looking forward to it because last time he couldn't keep up with her or walk around comfortably.

Don is looking into a morphine patch to help his pain, which is pretty much his last resort, but he needs to work on his attitude. Can a therapist help Don? Can his wife? Can this marriage be saved? His medical team might be able to deal with his pain, but no one can help Don with his mindset except himself. Plenty of help is out there in books, in counselors, in alternative measures, but Don needs to open a valve in his mind that might let in calmness and ultimately give him some relief. Only he can do it.

Stress brought about by peripheral neuropathy can make all facets of a patient's life tiresome on everyone. In one chapter of *Pain Survival Guide:*

How to Reclaim Your Life: A Practitioner's Handbook, by Dennis C. Turk with Elena S. Monarch,[1] the authors discuss the demoralizing nature of chronic pain. If sufferers feel the continuing search for an elixir to relieve their pain remains out of reach, there seems to be no hope. The authors write about the importance of "emotional resilience." When chronic pain leaves one feeling helpless and hopeless, depression can add to the mix. It is not surprising that the depression can, over time, spread to the caregiver and to others in the household.

On Wellness Routines

When I began this project, my neuropathy had been in hiding for quite a while. Except for an angry flare because of stress or the weather, it was dormant. Then, about a month into research, it came roaring back, and was almost as bad as in the early days. And I know why. I was paying little attention to:

- My diet
- Vitamins and supplements
- Exercise routine
- Spiritual visits to church (on a regular basis)
- Hobbies
- Friends (some of them)
- Volunteer jobs (some of them)
- Proper amount of sleep

I wasn't a complete hermit, but writing the book was so much fun and absorbed so many hours that I didn't have time to stay on course, health-wise. I was having such a rewarding experience. How could my feet throw a monkey wrench into my system and mess things up?

Why? Because I had stopped my own wellness routine, the one that works for me and for millions, whether they have neuropathy or not. What other reason could there possibly be for me to go downhill so quickly? I was forgetting to do those things so vital to wellness that I mentioned in the book! I was unconsciously letting things slide.

La-dee-dah. I can skip all that stuff, I told myself. But I *can't* skip all that stuff. And neither can you if you care about your health.

I am back now into my wellness routine, more or less, and my peripheral neuropathy is taking a back seat again. The hardest thing to ramp up is my walking. My mind is saying, "*How can you vigorously walk when your feet hurt so much?*" When I make myself walk despite the burning, my feet like it; the walking acts as a massage, and they don't bother me as much.

This is not an "alert the media" scientific experiment. I'm just telling you what happened when I became sloppy with my wellness plan, and how I got my mojo back.

The moral of the story is to never lose sight of your goals. At the risk of redundancy, think about proper nutrition and rest, intellectual nourishment, spiritual grounding, love for your passions, social connections, and volunteering. If you follow those pathways, wellness might not be around the corner; however, you will have the power and positive attitude to receive a sense of well-being. Although you can't cure or stop your neuropathy, you will make your life more enjoyable.

Life in a Minor Key

Sometimes when your life is played in a minor key,
the most wonderful things can happen. . . . Sometimes when you
get knocked down, you are better than you ever were.
—Pastor John Dolaghan, The Chapel at Sawgrass

If you feel that your life is played in a minor key because of your peripheral neuropathy, take heart in those words. Make them part of your very fiber. Take your health frustrations as an opportunity for growth, and turn your handicaps into opportunities.

You know a cure is out there. You need to be ready. When your doctor tells you about it, you will be toned in mind, soul, and body, and in the best possible shape to receive it into your life. Welcome Wellness! Today, a cure is in the ozone, tomorrow it will be sitting on your doorstep.

For Further Reading

1. Turk, Dennis C., and Elena S. Monarch. *Pain Survival Guide: How to Reclaim Your Life: A Practitioner's Handbook*. Washington, DC: APA Lifetools.

10

Managing Your Physician

Norman Latov

Our medical care system is in flux nowadays, and probably will continue to be so for some time. But regardless of whether your care is provided in an office or clinic setting, lasts for an hour or 15 minutes, is paid for directly or is covered by insurance, your interaction with your physician will continue to play an important role in determining the outcome of your illness. This is particularly true for neuropathy, as it is often a chronic condition that requires complex decision making as you proceed with the evaluation and treatment.

To begin with, find a physician you like and trust; otherwise, it is unlikely that you will follow his or her advice. The most meaningful word in medical care is "care." A caring physician is more likely to pay attention, and less likely to miss anything important. Some sensitivity is required of the patient as well, as, for example, complaining about your other physicians might be counterproductive if the person you're talking to thinks that she might be next.

An increasingly important element in the patient–physician relation is that of time. Physicians nowadays, by necessity or mandate, have less time to spend with each patient largely due to dictates of managed care. Given the time limitations, it becomes more important to focus the discussion on the information that is most relevant to the neuropathy. With that out of the way, there is then room for quality time or other inquiries.

When visiting a physician for the first time, you will be asked about your symptoms and medical history, undergo a neurological examination, and be referred for tests to identify the cause. The opinions and recommendations of previous physicians are of interest, but usually less important, as physicians are ethically and legally responsible for their own decisions and actions. Your physician is therefore likely to insist on eliciting the history anew, rather than relying on previous records, and to request that you repeat any tests in which the results are ambiguous. Accordingly, physicians don't generally feel obliged to go along with other physician's recommendations, if they do not agree with the assessment.

Having some general knowledge of neuropathy will help you understand what historical information is most relevant, and what to expect in the course of the interview and examination. It will also help you set realistic goals and expectations. It is beyond the scope of this book to delve into the various medical aspects of neuropathy, such as the explanation of the symptoms, causes, and available treatments, but you can find a relatively easy-to-understand discussion of these topics in my book *Peripheral Neuropathy: When the Numbness, Weakness and Pain Won't Stop*, part of the American Academy of Neurology Press Quality of Life Guide Series. The information will probably not be sufficient to allow you to diagnose your condition without a neurological evaluation, but it will help you understand what you're feeling, and to communicate more effectively with your physician.

Diagnosis

The most common cause of neuropathy is diabetes. Other than that, neuropathy can be caused by nutritional deficiencies, toxins, infectious agents, autoimmune diseases, cancer, or some hereditary disorders. In about one-third of cases, no cause can be found, in which case the neuropathy is called *idiopathic*, a not particularly helpful term that, according to Mims Cushing, is jokingly derived from the words *idiot* and *pathetic*.

To identify the cause of the neuropathy, a physician relies on the history, examination, and laboratory testing. The most important information that the patient provides is the history of the illness; the other two elements are elicited by the physician. The following is a listing of the information that your physician will find most relevant. You might consider printing it in succinct form and handing it to your physician at the time of your visit.

History

Onset
- What were the initial symptoms?
- When did they start?
- Which part of the body was initially affected?
- Did the symptoms begin suddenly or gradually?
- Were they preceded by an illness, food poisoning, vaccination, a new medication, travel, or exposure to a toxin? Were other people affected at the time?

- Were you drinking excessive amounts of alcohol, or eating a diet rich in fish that contain high mercury levels?

Current Symptoms

- Do you have weakness? If yes:
    - Is the weakness in the arms or legs, and in which muscles?
    - Do you have difficulty with walking, going up or down stairs, carrying packages, or turning a key?
- Do you have sensory symptoms? If yes:
    - Is it numbness, pain, or annoying sensations? Provide a succinct description.
    - Which parts of the body are affected; the legs, arms, torso, or face?
    - Are the symptoms constant or fluctuating, and are they more severe at night or aggravated by walking or other activities?
    - Do you feel pain if you accidentally stick yourself with a sharp object, or suffer a cut or a burn?
    - Do you have systemic symptoms such as dizziness or rapid heartbeat when standing up, abnormal sweating, frequent diarrhea or constipation, or fullness after eating small amounts of food?
- Do you have impaired coordination in the arms or legs? If yes:
    - Do you lose your balance easily, or fall?
    - Does your hand tremor when you use it?
    - Do you have difficulty with fine movements such as when buttoning your shirt?

Course

- Have the symptoms increased recently, improved, fluctuated, or stayed the same?
- What is the overall course of the illness since it began?
- Family history
- Has anyone else in your family been diagnosed with neuropathy, or have similar symptoms?

Other Medical Conditions
Some, such diabetes, could be the cause of the neuropathy.

Medications
List your current medications, and those that you were taking when the symptoms began, as certain medications can cause neuropathy.

Previous Evaluations

- If you have been previously evaluated, what were the results of the investigations?
  - Bring in copies of previous medical summaries, and reports of MRIs, EMG and nerve conduction studies, spinal taps, blood tests, or other relevant studies.
  - Don't assume that copies of your records will be forwarded to the office upon request, even if so promised. Our own success rate is approximately 50%. Pick these up yourself or have them mailed to you, and bring them with you to the visit. Keep a set for your records.
  - Look through the materials before the visit, to organize them by date or specialty, and remove duplicates, or irrelevant documents such as bills or unrelated medical reports. Most handwritten notes are unreadable. Time spent reviewing the records will take away from your time with the physician.
- Previous treatments? If yes:
  - Were you treated for the underlying cause of the neuropathy, and if so, when, with what procedure or medication, for how long, the dose, any side effects, and the results of each treatment?
  - Did you receive treatment for your symptoms, including for pain, and if so, when, with what medication or procedure, for how long, what was the dose, the side effects, and the results of each treatment?

Based on your responses, your physician might ask additional questions or request more detailed information regarding particular aspects of the history that could be relevant.

The Examination

The neurologic examination is rather standard and hasn't changed much since the 19th century. Its purpose is to identify the motor or sensory deficits, delineate the anatomical distribution, and quantify the severity.

Strength is routinely evaluated by manual muscle testing, or by testing such functions as walking on the heels or toes, getting up from a chair, or rising from a kneeling position without using your hands. Coordination and balance are evaluated by testing for repetitive or alternating movement of the hands or feet, touching the tip of the nose with the eyes closed, or walking heel-to-toe as if on a tightrope. Tapping with a rubber hammer is used to test for reflexes at the elbows, knees, and ankles.

Sensory functions in the hands and feet are evaluated by using a pin to test for pain perception, a tuning fork for vibratory perception, a warm or cold object for temperature sensation, or a cotton tip for perception of light touch. Position sense is tested by the ability to perceive up or down movements of the fingers or toes with your eyes closed.

The examination is often repeated at subsequent visits to help determine whether the neuropathy has progressed, improved, or stayed the same, based on changes in the neurological deficits. In the case of sensory neuropathy, in particular, the symptoms are not always a reliable measure of the severity of the underlying neuropathy. The pain can increase or decrease despite improvement or progression of the underlying neuropathy, due to hypersensitivity or replacement by numbness.

Laboratory Tests

If neuropathy is suspected based on the symptoms or examination, two types of tests are used to confirm the presence of, and delineate the extent of, the neuropathy.

If the neuropathy affects the large nerve fibers, the abnormalities can be detected and delineated by electromyography (EMG) and nerve conduction (NC) studies that measure the electrical properties of the nerves. The studies, in addition, provide information regarding whether the neuropathy primarily affects the nerve processes, called *axons*, or the *myelin sheath* that insulates the nerves. Some diseases preferentially affect one or the other, so that this information can provide a clue to the underlying cause.

Some neuropathies, however, affect only the small nerve fibers, so that the EMG and NC studies are normal. Small-fiber neuropathies can be very painful, but sometimes missed by physicians, as they often cause only subtle sensory deficits, and the neurological examination may be normal. Some of these patients may have been mistakenly told that they had fibromyalgia, reflex sympathetic dystrophy, or a psychiatric disorder before they were finally diagnosed with neuropathy. The diagnosis, however, can be made in a physician's office, by doing a 3-mm skin biopsy and demonstrating a reduction in the density of the skin or epidermal nerve fibers. The test is particularly useful in patients with unexplained pain syndromes, as many of these are caused by neuropathy. The skin biopsy can be repeated at a later time if there is question as to whether it has progressed, improved, or remained the same.

Once the presence of neuropathy is established, the physician will order a number of blood tests for possible causes, based on the characteristics of the neuropathy. If no cause can be found, the neuropathy is considered idiopathic, in which case it is usually treated symptomatically and followed by periodic examinations. If the neuropathy progresses, then the physician might recommend a nerve and muscle biopsy, as this type of examination of the damaged nerve can occasionally reveal a cause that was not identifiable through the other studies. The biopsy, however, can cause lingering pain in a small percentage of cases, so it not generally performed unless the neuropathy is progressive and the cause cannot be otherwise identified.

Treatment

Treatment is generally directed at both the underlying neuropathy and its symptoms. Treatment for the underlying neuropathy depends on the cause, as, for example, controlling the blood sugar in diabetes, or giving vitamin B_{12} shots for vitamin deficiency. The goal of such treatments is to prevent further damage and allow the nerves to heal. Peripheral nerves have a limited capacity to regenerate, however, so that recovery is often incomplete, and the symptoms could persist, although with variable degrees of improvement. The extent of recovery depends on the severity and type of damage that's already present, the ability to prevent further damage, and the nerve's capacity to heal. No medications currently are available that enhance nerve regeneration, but early intervention and treatment can limit the injury and optimize the chances for a more complete recovery.

Physical and occupational therapy can help maintain and improve motor functions, regardless of the severity of the neuropathy. A variety of medications are available for neuropathic pain, but no one medication works for everyone, so each patient has to determine his best regimen, based on trial and error. If standard treatments fail, your physician may refer you to a *pain center*, where more treatment options are available, and where the staff has greater expertise in managing acute and chronic pain. It is helpful to keep a log with a list of your daily medications, and to score the pain daily on a scale of 1–10. This could help you compare the effectiveness of the various medications as you determine the regimen that works best for you.

In recommending a particular treatment over another, a doctor usually takes into account such factors as the severity of the neuropathy, rate of progression, concurrent medical conditions, potential drug interactions, age, and susceptibility to developing particular side effects or adverse reactions. For example, the presence of glucose intolerance is a relative counter-indication to prednisone, as one of the potential side effects is diabetes. Your physician will want to discuss the various treatment options with you, before deciding on which to recommend.

Most doctors do not routinely prescribe alternative therapies, such as nutritional supplements, as there is no general agreement regarding when or how to use them, or whether they help at all. That's why they are considered alternatives. However, deficiencies of vitamin B_{12}, B_6, or B_1 can cause neuropathy, so blood levels are routinely tested in suspected cases, and supplements are prescribed if a deficiency is found. If a deficient diet is suspected, daily supplements of 1,000 mcg B_{12}, 50 mg B_1, and 50 mg B_6 are often recommended. Be careful not to take too much B_6, however, as excessive amounts can be toxic to nerves. Alpha lipoic acid, at doses of 600–800 mg/day, has traditionally been considered an alternative treatment, but more recent evidence that it may be helpful in diabetic neuropathy is slowly bringing it into the mainstream of medical treatments.

Last, but not least, consider making friends with the office staff. After all, they are the gatekeepers. If you decide to bring cookies, remember to bring enough for everyone, including other patients, but don't get the expensive kind, as you might run afoul of Medicare's anti-inducement statute.

11

Frequently Asked Questions

Norman Latov

1. If one has no open sore, is it safe to use soothing, over-the-counter creams on feet or hands?

Such creams are generally safe, so that having neuropathy is not a reason not to use them, if they are helpful.

2. Peripheral neuropathy used to be thought of as a "glove-and-stocking" problem that is, affecting the hands and feet, but it can affect so many other areas. Can you talk about these "other areas"?

"Glove-and-stocking" refers to a common pattern of involvement in polyneuropathy, as it often affects the hands and feet. This pattern is characteristic of "length-dependent" neuropathies that affect the most distal nerve segments first. In other, non–length-dependent neuropathies, however, other parts of the body can be affected, including the torso or face.

3. What has been discovered in the past 10 years in the way of treatment modalities, ways of screening, and other advances?

A number of gene defects that cause hereditary neuropathies were identified that can now be tested for, if suspected. Antiganglionic nicotinic acetylcholine receptor antibodies were discovered to cause an autoimmune autonomic neuropathy that can improve with therapy. Small-fiber neuropathy can now be diagnosed by skin biopsy and visualization of the epidermal nerve fibers. Lidoderm Patch (lidocaine 5%), Cymbalta (duloxetine), and Lyrica (pregabalin) were introduced for the treatment of diabetic neuropathic pain.

4. What is E-Stim and is it effective on peripheral neuropathy?

These are instruments that stimulate muscle contractions They help maintain muscle tone, but they do not increase strength, and have no direct effect on nerves.

5. Sciatica is a neuropathy problem that is very common. But I don't think people realize it is one of the peripheral neuropathy diseases. What other things are not usually linked with neuropathy but, in fact, are?

Sciatica is used to describe a pain syndrome that results from compression of the sciatic nerve in the lower back, with radiating pain down the leg. It's a *focal neuropathy* that results from local compression of a single nerve. Carpal tunnel syndrome, facial palsy, trigeminal neuralgia, and tarsal tunnel syndrome, among others, are other types of focal neuropathies.

6. It seems that you don't sweat in your lower extremities when you have nerve pain in your legs/feet. Does that make you sweat more in the head and face?

Sweating is a compensatory mechanism to cool the body when it is overheated. As the sweat glands in the skin are regulated by autonomic nerve fibers, those parts of the body that are affected by neuropathy lose the ability to sweat. When the legs are affected, other, unaffected parts of the body such as the skin or head sweat excessively to compensate.

7. Skin can be really sensitive after shingles. Does that go away?

After an acute attack of shingles, the nerve heals slowly, and may remain painful or sensitive for a long time. The sensitivity may eventually go away, but not always, depending on the extent of damage and regenerative capacity of the nerve.

8. Can borderline diabetes spark peripheral neuropathy?

Yes, it can. Some people with borderline diabetes are more susceptible to developing neuropathy than others, for reasons that we do not yet understand. Those who are more easily affected have to work harder at keeping the blood glucose levels in the normal range.

9. Can nerves heal over time?

To some extent, depending on the type and severity of the damage already present and ongoing disease activity. *Demyelinating neuropathies* heal more easily than axonal neuropathies, and mild neuropathies heal better than if severe damage is present. It is therefore important to treat early, to preserve function.

10. If the nerves in your feet have died, does that mean that you feel no more pain?

Not necessarily. The nerves usually extend from the spinal cord to the skin. Even if the distal parts are dead, the more proximal segments can generate pain signals.

11. So many prescription drugs have the qualifier "Not for everyone." How long should you stay with a med if you're having problems with it, such as weight gain, insomnia? Does that problem stop after a while, once your body gets used to the drug?

Both therapeutic benefit and side effects are usually dose dependent, so that if side effects occur at doses that are subtherapeutic, then they are unlikely to go away. At the onset, however, the metabolism can change as the body adapts to the new medication, so that it is advisable to introduce the drug at relatively low doses and increase it slowly, to maximize the chances of obtaining a therapeutic benefit without the side effects. How long you stay on any given medication before evaluating its therapeutic benefits depends on the individual medication. Your physician can assist you in this analysis.

12. Is it OK to use hot tubs or whirlpools at spas and clubs? Who can and who cannot use them?

It is usually OK, except with autonomic neuropathy that causes low blood pressure. The heat causes the blood vessels in the skin to dilate, so that blood is diverted to the skin from other parts of the body, including the brain. This is called *vasodilatation*. The effect is to lower the blood pressure further, resulting in dizziness or fainting Alcohol can also induce vasodilatation, and blood is diverted to the gut after eating, or to the muscles after exercise, so these can aggravate the fall in blood pressure.

13. How common are amputations with diabetic peripheral neuropathy (DPN)?

Amputations are uncommon, except in severe diabetic neuropathy. Diabetes also impairs circulation and immunity, as well as prevents healing, so that in cases of a severe infection, amputation may be necessary to prevent the spread of the infection to other parts of the body.

14. Does cutting the nerves ever help?

Rarely, as occasionally in the case of *neuroma*. However, if the pain signals are generated more proximally to the resection, cutting the distal part of the nerve won't help.

15. I've heard that orthotics can weaken muscle usage and that people should wait until they absolutely must have them before trying them. Your thoughts?

Orthotics are simply foot-supporting devices. The best time to begin using orthotics is when you need them to improve your function, such as the ability to walk. They don't have to be worn all the time, however, so that the muscles can still be used at times, preventing deterioration from lack of use.

16. When feet are roasting hot, is it all right to soak them in icy water?

Cooling the feet when they feel hot and burning can be soothing, but icy water can cause frostbite, especially if the neuropathy prevents you from feeling the cold. Better to use cold water without ice, or a refrigerated gel pack, and dry well afterward to avoid trench foot.

17. When some people cut out sugar, their peripheral neuropathy eases up. If they are not a diabetic, might that mean they could be in future?

Such people should be checked for a pre-diabetic condition called *glucose intolerance*, where the blood sugar levels stay up for too long after meals.

18. Are there statistics on what percentages of people (of the 20 million) have the various types of neuropathy (i.e., 25% have chronic inflammatory demyelinating polyneuropathy [CIDP], 10% have Guillain-Barré syndrome [GBS], etc.)?

Reliable numbers are not available, but it is thought that approximately 40% have diabetes, 20% inflammatory causes including CIDP and GBS, 15% nutritional, 10% hereditary, and 15% covers all the rest.

19. What kinds of neuropathy can you die from, if any?

Severe cases of GBS can be fatal, particularly if there is respiratory failure with pulmonary infection, or cardiac arrhythmias from autonomic involvement. *Amyloidosis* can also be fatal, as it can cause progressive autonomic failure. Neuropathies associated with tumors, such as lung cancer or myeloma, are not by themselves fatal, but the underlying tumor can be.

20. Many people with celiac disease have neuropathy. Should we all be eating gluten-free breads and pastas?

I often wondered whether people in the Far East live longer because they eat rice instead of bread, but there is no evidence that gluten is harmful if you do not have celiac disease.

21. I've heard several people say their electromyogram (EMG) tests showed that they have carpal tunnel, yet they have no pain. How is that explained?

Carpal tunnel syndrome (CTS) occurs when the median nerve is compressed at the wrist. The compression can be detected by EMG, and nerve conduction studies. In cases where the compression is mild, the carpal tunnel may be asymptomatic.

22. What is vasculitis, and how do you test for it? Is it considered a neuropathy?

Vasculitis is an inflammation of your blood vessels. *Vasculitic neuropathy* results from inflammation of the blood vessels in the nerves. The vasculitis can be restricted to the nerves, or systemic and affecting other organs, or associated with such conditions as polyarteritis nodosa or hepatitis C. If restricted to the nerves, nerve and muscle biopsy is usually required to make the diagnosis.

23. If one's peripheral neuropathy doesn't seem to have changed, should one still go to see his or her neurologist and, if so, how often?

Neuropathies can stabilize, with no further progression, in which case routine follow-up visits with the general physician would suffice. However, in some cases, such as painless sensory neuropathy. for example, it may be difficult to tell if there is progression, so it is important to see the neurologist first, and she can recommend further treatment.

24. What is IVIg? I've read that doctors don't really know how it works. Can you explain it?

IVIg stands for *intravenous gammaglobulins*. It was initially used to boost immunoglobulin levels in immune-deficient patients, but accidentally found to also have potent anti-autoimmune activity, including in

CIDP and GBS. A number of mechanisms of action have been proposed, but no one is sure which one is most important, so that is still a mystery. Consequently, some physicians consider it their own form of alternative therapy.

25. What is plasmapheresis? How does it work ... and *does* it work?

Plasmapheresis is like dialysis, but for large proteins. It is used to remove antibodies from the bloodstream, thereby preventing them from attacking their targets. It has been shown to be effective in CIDP and GBS, presumably by removing anti-nerve antibodies.

26. About Sjögren's syndrome: I always thought it was dry eyes and dry mouth, but I understand there are a lot of other parts of the body it can affect. Please discuss.

Sjögren's syndrome can also cause an inflammatory neuropathy, as well as chronic fatigue, arthritis, and other autoimmune syndromes. The neuropathy of Sjögren's syndrome is often sensory, and mostly affects the small fibers or the cell bodies of the sensory nerves. It is one of the most prevalent autoimmune disorders, affecting as many as 4 million Americans. You can contact the Sjögren's Syndrome Foundation to find out more about this condition.

27. I am hot from the knees up, but the calves of my legs are freezing, even when it's in the 70s in my house. Is that part of my sensory neuropathy?

Burning or freezing pains are types of spontaneous sensations, called *paresthesias*, that occur when the sensory nerves are damaged. They can also cause numbness, tingling, itching, stinging, buzzing, shooting, or electric-like sensations, among others. It may feel like there are different things going on in the body, but its all the same to the nerves.

28. Has any neuropathy study been made that asks questions about what people eat (or have eaten in the past) that may be causing their neuropathy? Examples: Did you use saccharin when it first came out in the '50s, and do you still use sugarless sweeteners? How many canned vegetables do you eat in a month? And so on.

There isn't much known about it, except that too much fish can cause mercury toxicity, a strict vegetarian diet often lacks vitamin B_{12}, and bread can aggravate celiac disease. People either didn't look very hard, or didn't find anything. However, it may also be that a great deal of variation exists between individuals, so that particular foods may affect different people in different ways.

29. What is *multifocal neuropathy*, and how does it differ from *polyneuropathy*?

Multifocal neuropathy is a descriptive term applied to neuropathies that affect some nerves but not others in a multifocal distribution. Polyneuropathy, on the other hand, affects all nerves relatively equally. Multifocal neuropathies are often caused by inflammatory conditions, whereas polyneuropathies can result from diffuse processes such as nutritional deficiencies or toxins.

30. What are your views on the flu shot?

It's a good idea in general. However, vaccination stimulates the immune system, so that if you have an autoimmune condition, a small chance exists that it might be aggravated by the vaccine. That being said, its best to get the vaccine if you have an underlying condition that would make getting the flu particularly dangerous, such as chronic pulmonary disease.

31. Loss of balance is common in aging and in peripheral neuropathy. How can one tell what it is from?

In neuropathy, lack of balance results from interference with sensory and motor signals that tell the brain where the feet are in space, or coordinate the movements of the muscles in the legs. Neuropathy can be tested for separately to see if it is present.

32. What part does attitude play in how well you can keep your peripheral neuropathy under control?

Attitude doesn't affect the neuropathy itself, but it is an important determinant in how you deal with it and how it affects your life.

33. Do statins cause neuropathy?

Statins can cause neuropathy, but they also save lives. If your neuropathy was aggravated or began soon after taking statins, you might consider discontinuing the medication for a period of about 3 months, to see if there is any improvement.

12

The Hope of Research

Norman Latov

For many people, coming to grips with neuropathy occurs through several stages. Initially, there is the anxiety and worry that comes with the realization that something is awry with your body. This typically begins a phase of trying to find out what is wrong and where to go for help. Then a period of intense activity occurs, going back and forth for tests, doctor appointments, learning about the diagnosis, and beginning treatment. Finally, there is a prolonged period of learning to live with a chronic illness and to manage symptoms that may never entirely go away. People get along as best as they can, ranging from poorly to pretty good, but life is never quite the same afterward.

The majority of people facing a chronic condition become complacent, feeling powerless and accepting their fate, as there is little they can do. Others, however, continue to fight; they join support groups or online communities, travel to health spas or medical centers, experiment with diets or alternative medicines, and take up tai-chi or yoga, to help strengthen their bodies and minds. Regardless of how successful these various techniques are by themselves, through these efforts it's possible to create a community of like-minded individuals, all reaching out for information and providing help, understanding, and support for one another.

It takes more than that, however, to find a cure. For, after all is said and done, the pain is too often still there, especially at night, in bed, when we're all alone. Believing that a cure can be found, however, requires faith, hope, and understanding. Faith in the ability of science to find and fix what is wrong, hope that a cure is on the horizon, and understanding that you can, in fact, help make that happen.

Most people think of research as something mystical, beyond their grasp or understanding. Although it is true that there is a language barrier that requires translation, the concepts themselves are rather simple and straightforward. The body is very much like a machine, similar to a car engine. If you can figure out how it works, and what went wrong, you can usually come up with a way to fix it. The tools may be different, in that you may use a microscope or test tube instead of a wrench or hammer, but you are still just looking to see where the problem lies. The knee is connected to the shin bone, the same way as the crankshaft is connected to a piston, and so on. This is how it works on a subcellular level as well.

The process of discovery in science is in many ways no different than in other human endeavors, like Columbus discovering the Americas, or Lewis and Clark the Northwest Passage. The tools and training may be different, but in all cases, the process requires an inquisitive spirit, aided by persistence, insight, brilliance, and serendipity. The more people who are out there looking, and in more places, the better the chances that something important will be discovered.

Research is expensive, but the total amount is miniscule compared to the cost of the disease burden itself. For example, just the cost of intravenous immunoglobulin (IVIg) for treating Guillain-Barré syndrome and chronic inflammatory demyelinating polyneuropathy (CIDP) is probably more than ten times the annual research budget of the National Institutes of Health (NIH) for all the different types of neuropathy combined. At the same time, hardly any grants for finding the cause of these diseases have been awarded in the past 10 years. Just think of what might have happened if the money that went into polio research was all spent on buying iron lungs instead of also for developing a vaccine.

In the United States, medical research is largely funded by the NIH. Where that funding is directed is important, not only because it pays for research directly, but because it also determines the priorities of the medical academic centers that increasingly rely on that revenue stream. This applies not only to their research agendas, but also to their clinical and training programs, as many of the same faculty are active in all three spheres. Without NIH funding, there is then little interest in developing neuropathy research or clinical programs, or in teaching about neuropathy to medical students. This sets up a downward spiral, because with fewer academicians working on neuropathy, there is less interest in the subject among members of NIH grant review committees and fewer grants awarded for neuropathy at the next funding cycle. However, we live in a participatory democracy, so that we need to speak up, organize, and participate if we want neuropathy research to get its fair share.

We can also help by donating to laboratories that do research in neuropathy. This can be done directly, or through organizations that award research grants. With approximately 20 million people in this country suffering from neuropathy, if we each made a small donation, it would quickly add up to a very large sum. With everyone joining in the effort, neuropathy would have nowhere to hide.

13

Peripheral Neuropathy Stories by Those Who Know It Best

Mims Cushing

The one who tells the stories rules the world.
—Hopi

If you have read the tips and are still not convinced that *You CAN Cope with Peripheral Neuropathy*, then try reading the following stories by people who are, indeed, coping with it.

These stories are inspiring because the authors have battled ignorance, struggled to gain knowledge, and are living their lives with grace. The stories describe both fairly easy-to-manage types of neuropathy, as well as more complicated ones requiring special treatments.

Perhaps you will see yourself in one of these stories. Maybe you are a pregnant mother and have neuropathy. Terry Rees had peripheral neuropathy when she was pregnant at age 22 in 1964. Were you in the service in Vietnam, and exposed to dioxin? Read Eugene Richardson's story. It took him decades to be properly diagnosed. Maybe you have a young child with neuropathy. Shane Gibbs started on his neuropathic journey at age 6. When she was a child, Bev Anderson had trouble playing sports—peripheral neuropathy was the problem, but she didn't know it. Perhaps you have a child who has an awkward time with sports. Could it be peripheral neuropathy? It could.

Welcome these writers. Read, digest, and metabolize their stories. Their writings are gifts to you from them, and they are cheerleading for you.

Meet Howard

Howard Ettlinger, 70, and I were discussing the phrase "boy toy." He said, "You can call me a boy toy, but Mattel would probably say I need to be recalled." He tells me he is "working like a dog." He sells dozens of his creative trinket boxes through ads in a newsletter that circulates in his apartment building. Some days, his hands are so bad he can't hold a fork, but when he wants to make boxes or pillows, God lets his hands work. Along with his walker and crutches, he stores many of his creations in one shower in his apartment. "Don't write 'bathtub,'" he says. "It makes me think of bathtub gin."

"Howard, how do you cope?" I asked. In a hushed voice, as though it's the secret of the century he tells me, "I found something new: *vodka*! I drink it as I watch Oprah at 4:00 p.m., and then I go and have a nice dinner."

A Healthy Body and Good Mental Health Go Hand in Hand
by Howard Ettlinger

*Before I learned how to cope with neuropathy, or even knew what it was ... well, let's go back to the beginning, even before my trip to the Emerald City to see the Wizard. (*The Wizard being a "second-opinion doctor" at the University of Florida-Shands Hospital in Gainesville. MC*) It all started 20 years ago with the first of my 15 foot surgeries. My foot never healed. I was always coming down with infections—I do not have diabetes—and one day my foot doctor in Jacksonville told me I had to have my right leg amputated below the knee.*

He recommended a foot surgeon at Shands-Gainesville, so I had a half-hour visit with him, and he said I had neuropathy. Returning to Jacksonville, I went to another doctor to treat me for an open wound, but it was always getting infected. That doctor got together with an infectious diseases doctor, and they decided I needed to have a toe amputated, which I agreed to.

An open wound on the bottom of my foot has gone through five skin grafts (no pain involved). It's not healing because of the neuropathy. The wound is just about closed, and I may not need another graft.

My neuropathy has no known cause. Years ago, I went to a support group. I thought I was the only one with this illness, and then heard others speak about their problems. I found out there is no cure, but I heard about a drug that many were taking, and I told my foot doctor about it, and it worked for a while. I also learned to sleep with socks. It's supposed to quiet down the neuropathy, perhaps tell it to go to sleep, and it works somewhat.

When I was asked to write this piece about how I cope, I thought about the Holocaust and what the people did to survive. I don't think about what I do to survive. I am in charge of my neuropathy, and not the other way around. I'm like the Energizer Bunny. I just keep goin' and goin'. . . .

When we have quiet time in church, my body feels more relaxed and free of pain, so why can't I do that at home? I recently moved and, in my little study, I sit in my chair and watch the planes take off from NAS Jax (the Naval Air Station in Jacksonville, Florida) *and something happens that lets me feel calm.*

When I worked prior to the year 2000, I popped pain pills and would lie on the floor crying hysterically. I underwent plasmapheresis, in which a person's blood plasma is removed and then replaced with a synthetic substitute. I had to lie there for hours. What it had to do with my neuropathy, I have no idea. It was torture.

That seems like 100 years ago. Today, I'm by no means pain free, and the bottom of my foot still has not completely healed because of the neuropathy, but I've gone from a 10 plus (on a pain scale) to maybe a 2 or 3. I know what to do when the pain comes, and that is to look out the window, or shut my eyes and take myself to a happy place, of which I have many. I think of myself as a cloud or a bird, and I'm sailing through the sky without pain. Even the scent of a cologne or perfume can start my trip. I also listen to meditation tapes. It took me a long time to figure out how helpful they are.

I was doing okay today until 5:00 P.M., but I had dinner to finish so I put the pain out of my mind and told it to come back later. It hasn't returned, so maybe it got lost. I had spare ribs, corn, cauliflower, and roasted potatoes. Now I can get me a piece of apple pie with whipped cream. When I tell you I don't know why I can't lose weight, remind me of what I just ate for dinner. This story of my peripheral neuropathy is my gift to you.

Remember, you are the travel agent and can take yourself wherever you want to go. Go back as far as you want in time, or jump ahead. Doctors can help, but you are in control over your body and what happens to it.

— HOWARD ETTLINGER

Meet Fred

When Fred Roberts walked into a support group meeting in Florida in 2001, I thought, "What a good looking guy." He impressed me with his attitude: always upbeat. His peripheral neuropathy started in the 1980s, when he noticed numbness in his toes. I talked to him recently on the telephone, and he told me his story.

A Positive Attitude Gets Him Dancing
by Fred Roberts

Numbness bothered me in the mid-80s, and the sensation was constant. My wife back then said, "I think you have neuropathy." Well, I saw one doctor who did the electrical conduction studies, then I went to another. And had it done all over again with a third doctor, and that's no fun, but I wanted a third opinion. All of them agreed. It was peripheral neuropathy.

I worked on the waterfront with the International Longshoremen's Association, working on the docks as well as doing paper work and directing the loading of container ships. Because I had lost a good deal of my balance, and because I had had a stroke, I went on disability at the age of 60. My wife died right around that time.

Today, I'm happy to say I go ballroom dancing every Friday at a singles dance club with my lady friend, whom I've been with for four years. Pretty good for 77.

I get iffy with ladders. I do a death grip on them and am getting numbness in my hands. They go to sleep real easy. Also, my neuropathy goes up my calves. I still use green aloe for the stinging and burning.

If your neuropathy allows you to do something you love, do it!
If not, find something you can do, and maybe
you will end up loving it.
—FRED ROBERTS

Meet Bev

Bev Anderson is a whirlwind, despite her foot woes. I believe she will not rest until every person in California is within striking distance of a peripheral neuropathy support group. Her organization, The Northern California Chapter of The Neuropathy Association, has achieved tax-exempt status—an arduous process. She encourages group leaders, finds lecturers for meetings and, in short, is 100% dedicated to the neuropathy cause. Bev grew up with her neuropathy (or perhaps neuropathy grew up with her).

Growing Up with Neuropathy
by Bev Anderson

It was always a mystery to me why other children could do simple things I could not. I was seen as clumsy. I perfected the art of falling.

It wasn't until high school, when I could take swimming most of the year, that I felt comfortable in a physical education class. I could run, but not with the speed or grace of others. Tracking an incoming softball was almost impossible. Playing basketball, I could drop the ball in the basket if I stood still, but if I ran and tried to keep my eyes on a ball, it proved disastrous. I could not roller skate, though I tried. Wearing heels was challenging, and often landed me on the floor. One never knows how another person's feet feel, but I knew mine were not the same as others. My feet have always had some numbness, but how do you know this if you've never had normal feeling? I amazed other teens when I ran barefoot across the hot blacktop and did not scream in pain when the temperature soared above 100. On the other hand, if I stepped on a pebble or puncture vine, that would cause much pain.

Being a Campfire Girl was special to me, but camp was a challenge. Long hikes caused pain. We'd come to a stream and others would balance well on a board or a path of stones across it. I'd step into the water not realizing I walked by sight, watching the water not the pathway. Night hikes with dim lights scared me, as I had little ability to know the lay of the land. My lack of reflexes also contributed to my lack of coordination. Walking a balance beam in class was necessary for teaching credentials. I cringed at my ineptness. Days of watching others climb a steep slope or scale a tree made me wonder: Why did my feet refuse to do what others could?

In high school, when I joined friends window shopping, I experienced my greatest pain. I remember standing in a store with tears running down my face, steeling myself to go on so I could keep up with my friends. I mentioned my problems to a doctor, and he said, "Oh, those are just growing pains." I knew plenty of people who were growing, but none of them had pain like I had. Once a friend said, "I always know it is you, Bev, because no one else walks like you do."

It wasn't until past middle adulthood that my little brother and I found we had something in common. We had never thought of comparing how we felt doing physical activity. He was diagnosed first. A year or so later, after I retired from 34 years of elementary school teaching, so was I. A neurologist told me to walk barefooted down a long hall, standing on my heels and then on my toes. I couldn't do it. He said, "I knew it was peripheral neuropathy when I saw you go down the hall. Diagnosis is easy. You have the 'neuropathy walk.'"

My brother and I knew our mother and maternal grandfather had the same complaints, and that we had had this from infancy. I especially walked like my grandfather. My brother's neuropathy was much worse than mine. I was determined to keep active and not let it affect my life as it did his.

Before he died of liver cancer, we agreed that neither of us having children was a blessing. We didn't want our children to suffer with something we passed along to them. Given that it hadn't skipped a generation, it was pretty much a sure thing that they, too, would have had neuropathy.

My counsel is to be aware that children can have peripheral neuropathy. A child who has difficulty with balance or is fearful in physical activity should be evaluated. I don't know that anything could have been done to change things or if knowing I had it would have made me think I should be less active. It might, however, have been reassuring to know I had a reason for my foot and balance problems. If people know they have a hereditary type of neuropathy, they might want to consider whether or not to have a child, just as they would if they had any other heredity disease. That's just my opinion.

Now, at 72, my sensory autonomic neuropathy is usually not as painful as earlier—or maybe I've gotten used to being in chronic pain. I don't spend much time sitting except for the hours I spend at the computer. I do physical activity in spurts, because being on my feet for a long stretch can be tiring and painful. In addition to being involved with my church, I spend a sizable amount of time developing The Northern California Chapter of The Neuropathy Association. My goal is to develop support groups throughout Northern California, so there is one within driving distance of everyone suffering from peripheral neuropathy. You can check our website at www.pnhelp.org to follow our progress.

> My counsel is to be aware that children can have
> peripheral neuropathy. A child who has difficulty with
> balance or is fearful in physical activity
> should be evaluated.
> — BEV ANDERSON

Meet Ron

A third of PNers have diabetic neuropathy, but two-thirds do not. So, it shouldn't be surprising that the majority of contributors to this chapter have neuropathy because of other causes. Ron has borderline diabetes.

Just Inside the Envelope
by Ron Gedney

My biggest frustration was trying to find out why my feet were going numb. My doctors in Virginia couldn't figure it out. Eventually we moved, and I saw a neurologist in New Smyrna Beach, Florida, who told me I had neuropathy. A neurosurgeon just spread his arms and said there was nothing he could do. I went to a podiatrist who arranged special inserts, but they just made my shoes too tight, and they did nothing for my neuropathy.

Independently, I found John Senneff's book, Numb Toes and Aching Soles.[1] *That book, as well as the website on neuropathy, were very helpful. For 5 years, the numbness was in my toes, then gradually encompassed the balls of both feet.*

As I am a borderline diabetic, staying just inside the envelope, I have substituted Splenda for sugar, which has brought down my blood sugar and seems to have slowed my neuropathy. In fact, in the last 3 years, it has hardly progressed at all,

Luckily, my neuropathy doesn't give me a lot of pain. Sometimes I can get along with no medication. If I don't wear shoes, I don't need meds, but when I do have to wear them, I need some pain relief. It helps to wear shoes that are loose, so they do not put pressure on my feet.

I do have discomfort. I feel as though I am getting electric shocks periodically, and my feet burn after I have walked short distances. Side effects of my peripheral neuropathy meds include muscle cramps and dizziness, but that could be due to my blood pressure medication.

I've discovered a treatment offered by physical therapists called Anodyne Therapy. For me, it seems to stimulate the blood flow to the foot, and it provides relief that lasts for a few hours. I put this on for 30 minutes, and my feet will be fine when I am trying to sleep, then I am good for the rest of the night. Of course, it doesn't always work.

No cause has been found for my neuropathy. Right now, all doctors can do is to treat the symptoms.

You can never go wrong if you cut back on sugar—
whether you have neuropathy or not.
—RON GEDNEY

Meet Eugene

On April 10, 2004, a miracle ended Eugene Richardson's 34-year-long nightmare. Since 1969, no doctor could diagnose or treat him. All those years when he became increasingly disabled, he was a successful senior career officer in the Army and then a vice president of operations in a private company. His strength and courage are inspiring to all in the Neuropathy Association support groups he heads in Broward and Highland Counties, Florida. He also lectures throughout the state for The Neuropathy Association and for groups sponsored by the Guillain-Barré–Chronic Inflammatory Demyelinating Polyneuropathy (GBS-CIDP) Foundation.

Coping Before the Miracle
By Lt. Col. Eugene B. Richardson, USA Retired

My symptoms began a year after I returned from Vietnam in 1968. For more than three decades, I lived with severe spinning sensations, breathing problems, and with chest muscles that did not work correctly, digestive problems, urinary incontinence, bouts of sweating, temporary chest paralysis, horrible electrical shocks, paralysis in my legs, and loss of sensation in my hands, feet, and eventually everywhere, as though a dentist had shot my body full of Novocain. I could not get a proper diagnosis.

Finally, my neurologist started me on intravenous gamma globulin (IVIg). Today, I take this intravenous drug every 21 days. I am disabled by CIDP, peripheral autonomic neuropathy, chronic sensory axonal polyneuropathy, and progressive polyneuropathy.

Extreme fatigue and muscle weakness ended my military career in 1989. Rumors were that it was all mental—the death knell for any military career officer. In the 1990s, my second career as a vice president came to a screeching halt because of bouts of temporary paralysis, breathing issues, and other symptoms. My CEO believed it was because I worked too hard.

Sometimes I agreed with doctors who said I was crazy. I feared I had a psychosomatic illness or a serious mental problem. I never knew when I might not be able to move, stand, sit, or walk. By the year 2000, I could no longer work. It was as though demons were playing in my body and mind, and no one could help me. I kept smiling and trying to hide my symptoms. Even so, people thought I was crazy, and who was I to disagree?

Finally, in 2000, a doctor said, "You have peripheral neuropathy." He listened. His words drove me into seeking information. Knowledge became the foundation for my strength in the face of a long journey. I didn't expect to find the negative attitudes, ignorance, and bias against those with peripheral neuropathy.

During those three decades without answers and, frankly, with incorrect conclusions from medical authorities, all I had was a belief in myself, my knowledge, my skills, and the support of my wife, Joyce, my many military friends, my pets, and my faith in God that someday the answer would be found. I believed that what my body told me was in opposition to everything doctors kept telling me. Often, humor got me through. When a neurologist scoffed, "Why do you need the cane?" I was shocked, but recovered to tell him I had it to eat in case I had to sit for hours in his waiting room and got hungry.

My pattern did not fit the textbooks. Doctors kept stating, "All tests are normal." I had an abnormal electromyogram (EMG)/nerve conduction test in 2000 that several doctors ignored. They didn't see the myelin damage. A doctor wrote, "Patient is claiming to have something he does not have." I crashed emotionally. In crying out to The Neuropathy Association staff, I received a phone call around midnight from the late Mary Ann Donovan, my angel in the night. She became my "go to" person.

For 4 more years, I went downhill. My nerves were severely damaged. Doctors tried to "make me" a diabetic, trying to mold me into a "textbook case." Finally, I was armed with a copy of the 2003 research provided by the 22-member medical advisory board of The Neuropathy Association. My neurologist read it and decided to do a trial of gamma globulin. My positive response confirmed his new suspicion of CIDP.

As symptoms abated after treatment with this intravenous product derived from human blood plasma (IVIg), I got up out of the wheelchair and could walk. Yes, my legs seemed to be made of rubber balloons and thick rubber, but I could walk, breathe, and talk at the same time.

Knowledge is the key to coping with this disease. You must become involved and be an advocate for yourself, no matter how threatened your doctor is of your involvement.

It soon became obvious that this miracle plasma product, IVIg, was not a simple one to administer. By listening to other patients, I learned what should be done, regarding the issues of correct administration of the product.

Once I landed in the ER struggling with pain, unable to walk, breathe, or talk because Medicare changes left me without the product: hospitals ran out of it. It was only because my wife found it at one hospital after 2 weeks of calling around. My doctor says I cheat death because of the IVIg.

In 2005, my legs turned into cement up to my waist because a VA doctor told me I could walk without the wheelchair and I wanted to believe him, but he was wrong. I needed an electric scooter. I must rest every 2 hours to avoid exhaustion. I can get around in the house and take out my best friend, my dog Bear, several times a day. Morning is best. The air is cool, the birds sing. . . .

These days, I focus on throwing myself into helping others and writing. My quest for knowledge has become an obsession. The Neuropathy Association's Neuropathy News newsletter is a lifeline for patients. It's where I found out I was not crazy. My outreach with newsletters to members gives meaning to my suffering and a focus that has strengthened my determination to help the cause of The Neuropathy Association.

A Special Note to Veterans
From Lt. Col. Eugene B. Richardson, USA Ret.

You served your country and have developed neuropathy (which has been diagnosed or not diagnosed) because of your service in a war zone where dioxin (Agent Orange) was used. I have heard the stories and read about the patterns of insidiously developing chronic and autonomic neuropathies told by thousands of veterans. My story is similar. I waited 34 years for a diagnosis and treatment—almost died in the process—but you know what? We are still here, and the courage endures. The good news is that we are still alive.

STEP ONE is to understand the good news. So, if you are reading this, the good news is that, in spite of your disabilities, you are ALIVE.

STEP TWO is to read this book for clues that may work for you and will help you live in spite of the effects of neuropathy on your body and your life.

STEP THREE is to read Dr. Norman Latov's book *Peripheral Neuropathy: When the Numbness, Weakness and Pain Won't Stop*, published in 2007. It is a wealth of knowledge from a man who cares.

STEP FOUR is to locate a board-certified neurologist who is trained in neuromuscular neurology and seek his help in four areas:

- To provide you with affirmation and a diagnosis for your chronic neuropathy (symptoms that last more than 60 days) or polyneuropathy (which affects many parts of your body) and possible treatment with gamma globulin.

- To work with you toward effective pain management, if present. Chronic pain must be treated.

- To rule in or out all known causes for your neuropathy and determine if your symptoms are supported by known patterns of the assumed cause.

- After all known causes are ruled out, to work to establish that there is a greater than 50% chance that your chronic neuropathy began as an acute neuropathy due to toxic exposure and then progressed to a chronic neuropathy. (See Citation Nr: 0306225: Decision Date: 04/01/03: Docket No. 97-18 169 on appeal from the Department of Veterans Affairs Regional Office in Milwaukee, WI. The Issue: Entitlement to Service Connection for Peripheral Neuropathy as a Result of Exposure to Agent Orange, see www.va.gov/vet/appo3/files/0306225.txt.)

STEP FIVE is to contact one of the organizations listed below and ask how to get in touch with a local Service Officer to help you apply for service-connected disability, based on your diagnosis of a peripheral neuropathy:

- Disabled American Veterans at www.dav.org
- Veterans of Foreign Wars at www.vfw.org

Or contact your local VA organization.

The fact that dioxin causes peripheral neuropathy has been well established scientifically. My neurologist has concluded, given that all causes and disease processes have been ruled out over four decades of testing, that my current diagnosis and symptoms are consistent with a toxic neuropathy due to dioxin exposure in the Vietnam War.

Neuropathy is an illness I would never choose; it was forced on me many years ago. Today, peripheral neuropathy is a worldwide enemy to millions and millions of people. My new mission is to find ways to live with it, teach others about it, and support efforts for a cure. The mission is a big one, but together we can win over neuropathy.

Someone once said to me, "How could you give hope and encouragement to someone? You're in a wheelchair." I responded, "The wheelchair is my strength; not my weakness.

—EUGENE RICHARDSON

Meet Tommy

If ever a man lived with good cheer all his life, it was Tommy McLaughlin, of Orange Park, Florida. Even after he was diagnosed with neuropathy, he was a pleasure to be around and loved by all, especially by his Jacksonville support group. I talked with his wife, Lorraine McLaughlin, and we put this together for you. —Mims Cushing

"It's a Lovely Day, Begorrah!"
Tommy McLaughlin's Story
By Lorraine McLaughlin, as told to Mims Cushing

It was a wasp nest that made Tommy McLaughlin realize something was wrong. He took his ladder, as he had many times, and climbed onto the roof of his home to attack the nest, but on that day something peculiar happened: He couldn't get down. "I was worried," said his wife, Lorraine, who was inside. "Tommy had been out there for 30 minutes." She went to look for him.

"I don't have the strength to get down," Tommy said. "I don't think I can keep my balance." She cheered him on—there wasn't much else she could do—and eventually he climbed down, slowly, his muscles weak, his balance off-kilter.

He didn't do anything about it, but in the following weeks, he'd tell Lorraine his feet were numb and he had no feeling in his legs. They had no idea what it was, but Tommy never dwelled on his pains.

About a year later, when he was 60, his feet felt as though he was walking on glass. He was a design engineer for the lumber industry and traveled all over the United States. He still didn't take his pains seriously and kept on working. Finally, he saw a doctor who told him he had peripheral neuropathy and gave him a pain prescription.

Lorraine says "We still had a wonderful time vacationing all over Europe with Tommy driving. He'd say, 'If we are going forward, I know my foot's on the accelerator. If we are stopped, it must be on the brake.' By this time, his feet were completely numb." It was time for a wheelchair, which prevented them from doing something they adored: dancing. "When he got a hold on you, you danced! I burned more dinners because he'd want me to stop everything and jitterbug or waltz. We won prizes when we were young."

He began going to a neuropathy support group in 1999, and everyone took an instant liking to him and Lorraine. She became the keeper of the name tags. She remembers, "Tommy greeted the

members with a twinkle in his eye and he would say, 'Top o' the mornin' to yah!' in that fake Irish brogue."

Tommy didn't retire until he was 75. He was always ready to have fun and ignore his pain. Finally, they bought a van with a lift. When his support group visited him in the hospital with cake and balloons, the members cheered him up and he encouraged them.

In 2005, Tommy died of lung cancer at the age of 80. Lorraine says the nurses and doctors loved him and, even today, she will be stopped by someone who says, "You're Tommy's wife! What a wonderful person he was. Doctors in the hospitals would say, 'Go into Tommy's room and you'll come out laughing.'"

Lorraine says, "The two of us were married for 60 years and rarely disagreed. Those who remember him will always think of his good cheer, even in the face of great pain."

Tommy felt his neuropathy was just one of those things. He just coped with it. And sometimes that's just what you have to do.
—LORRAINE MCLAUGHLIN

Meet Robert

Bob is another support group leader whom members are lucky to have. He hails from Virginia Beach, Virginia, and has added to the tips noted here and there in *Cope*. He has had his neuropathy for 33 years, and is 85 years old. This piece might be of interest if you are considering wearing orthotic braces.

A Work in Progress: Learning to Adapt
By Robert M. Williamson

I have never been known to rush into things, and my peripheral neuropathy has been right in character. My toes started feeling fuzzy in 1975, when I was 52 years old. I didn't report this to my primary care physician until 1981. Luckily, he was well informed and packed me off to a neurologist, who saw nerves in both legs responded poorly to generous electrical jolts. As no cause was found, I went my "idiopathic way," idiopathic meaning physicians haven't a clue.

I did know my increasing clumsiness was due to my underachieving sensory leg nerves. It was increasingly difficult to keep my balance. I had no pain, just numbness—a sensation that felt as though I was continuously wearing a stocking. I was heartened by the fact that this wasn't fatal—I would die with it, not from it.

*Long-term care insurers, however, do not look kindly on a poten-
tially debilitating disease, whether you die with it or from it.*

*Before long, my shoes began slapping on hard floors, and I
found myself stumbling and falling. Walking shoes with rocker bottom soles helped. In 1988, I quit playing tennis. Why didn't my neurologist tell me that "foot slap" and "foot drop" were caused by loss
of the motor nerves that control ankle muscles? Because I didn't tell
him my symptoms. Rather than complain, I took misguided pride
in being able to fall without breaking any bones. I know now that
drop foot is easy to identify: Lift a foot up off the floor. If you can't
keep it from rotating downward at the ankle, you have drop foot.*

*Because I couldn't balance well enough to bicycle on a two-
wheeler, I bought myself a stationary one. My leg strength didn't
improve, but I hoped I might be slowing the muscle decay. When no
cancer symptoms appeared, I quit worrying about that as a possible
cause of my peripheral neuropathy.*

*I finally became an unabashed user of foldable aluminum
canes. Although one suffices if I walk carefully, I need two when I
want to walk without fear of falling. One cane is always in front to
prevent me from falling forward. I use a shoulder bag or small
knapsack to carry things. Two canes provide a walking rhythm and
good arm exercise. I used to tell people I was getting in shape for
cross-country skiing, but that fib hasn't worked for years. Two canes
are a great help on uneven ground, on a short flight of stairs, or
when standing in a crowd.*

*In 1992, I met a person wearing short leg braces, ankle-foot-
orthotics (AFOs), and realized they were the answer to foot drop.
An AFO is a plastic brace, worn inside the shoe, that starts just
behind the ball of the foot and runs up the back of the leg to a strap
around the calf. My neurologist wrote a prescription, and an orthotist correctly judged that the lightest, pre-shaped AFO would do.
AFOs can also be custom-molded. Orthotists, podiatrists, and physical therapists are good judges of what kind of AFOs one needs.
After the first day, I was ready to toss the braces in the trash can.
They hurt my feet and cut into my calves.*

*After three trips back to the orthotist, who filed and reshaped
them and added wide leg straps, they worked well and continue to
do so. I use soft insoles in my shoes to cushion my feet, and that's
sufficient. I don't have to wear thick socks. I've learned it's good to
avoid AFOs as long as you can, because your muscles stiffen up
from inaction when you start wearing them, but at some point you
may have to.*

Light AFOs keep your feet from rotating downward at the ankles. Heavier ones provide lateral bracing. Both kinds improve your balance because some of the forces normally sensed by your feet are transmitted to sensory nerves in your calves. I avoid inside-the-shoe braces with devices that include narrow straps that run upward from your front shoelace holes to your lower legs. While these may prevent foot drop, they do not balance or provide bracing.

Prior to 2000, I was busy teaching physics and doing other teacher-related activities. When I moved to Virginia Beach and was fully retired, I became involved with our local peripheral neuropathy support group. I wondered if my first neurologist had tried hard enough to find the cause of my peripheral neuropathy. To my dismay, I found he had retired, and copies of the tests were no longer available. I now ask for copies of all medical tests and keep them on file at home.

My symptoms and their slow progress suggest that I may have a form of hereditary neuropathy for which no genetic markers have yet been identified. While I know of no peripheral neuropathy in my background, I can't be sure. Peripheral neuropathy was rarely diagnosed in the past. Elderly people shuffle and have balance problems for a variety of reasons.

I've complained for years about cold and somewhat discolored feet. Blood pressure checks along my legs show no circulation problem. Malfunctioning autonomic nerves that control capillary blood flow in the lower leg may be the cause of my symptoms. So, perhaps I'm a walking example of all three kinds of neuropathy in one body—sensory, motor, and autonomic. But I'm well aware of my good fortune in not having to contend with pain.

I taught college physics until retiring in 1991 and led teaching workshops until 2000. I could still walk short distances with care, without a cane. I had no trouble single-handling my small sailboat, but I sold it in 2006, as getting in and out had become too, let's just say, difficult. It's hard to tell whether my increasing leg weakness and fatigue are due to neuropathy, old age, or both. Whatever the cause, taking a nap after lunch helps.

Now, in 2008, I can still drive cars as long as they have big, well-spaced brake and accelerator pedals. The sensory nerves in my knees give me enough information to do this safely. I can't rotate my foot at the ankle, but I can exert downward force with the front of my foot. The AFO helps. I expect to get hand controls for my car or stop driving in another year or so. I gave up long ago trying to predict the rate of nerve decay or its final form.

I attempt a few steps without a cane only where there's a nearby object to grab in a pinch. My ankle muscles are useless, but my knees still work, and I can climb stairs if they have railings.

In summer, I swim in a pool with steps and a railing. I still manage air travel by myself. I volunteer as a docent at a Coast Guard Life Saving Station Museum. My wife and I enjoy local concerts and museums, where my rollator with a seat is invaluable. We take modest car trips and do Elderhostel adventures that include only limited walking.

And what of my hands? My fingers feel fuzzy. I need a puller for shirt buttons. I can barely tie shoe laces. In the old days, I haunted hardware stores looking for new shop tools. Now, I frequent medical supply stores and look through catalogs for "aids to living," such as key twisters and sock pullers. A slight hand tremor has given me an excuse for penmanship that has been illegible for years. I can, however, type with two fingers and that's how I am recording the ways I've coped. I hope this account of some of my mistakes and solutions will be helpful.

I was determined to keep on walking and did so regularly even though my legs felt dead due to the weakened leg muscles.

—ROBERT M. WILLIAMSON

Meet Irene

Ask anyone at The Neuropathy Association, and they'll tell you Irene Beer is the Association's most valued volunteer. She has pointed dozens of new support group leaders in the right direction, and is a support group leader herself. She is a frequent contributor to and co-editor of the *Neuropathy News* newsletter.

Irene has CIDP. For 11 years she has had IVIg treatments; nowadays, she is weaker in her thighs and lower legs and must use a cane.

From her homes in New York and Florida, she goes to PT and recently OT, as the neuropathy has gone into her hands. Irene's volunteering has deep roots. Here's what she tells us about the value of volunteering.

A Chronic Volunteer
By Irene H. Beer

When my neuropathy was first diagnosed in 1996, I was as confused as most people. I could not think straight. There was nowhere to turn, so I tried the Internet, but I didn't understand much of what I read.

Fortunately, here in New York, Dr. Norman Latov held a meeting to announce that Mary Ann Donovan would head a newly formed Neuropathy Association. I spoke to Mary Ann and said I wanted to volunteer, and we became good friends. I started volunteering right away and still do. I learned early on that knowledge is power.

I have always liked to assist in projects that interested me. In college, I worked as a camp counselor for physically handicapped children for five summers. I learned to help children realize their strengths in the pool. They acted in plays, went on local walks, and sang camp songs. I saw how doing things—rather than lying down and doing nothing—helped them cope. Those summers inspired me to go into the field of Special Education, working with physically handicapped children.

I also learned to cope with my own physical limitations and, when I developed neuropathy, I learned you can do anything you want. I thank all the people who have been there for me when I needed help.

Coping for me is learning about the situation, understanding what I have to do and how I can do it. . . and then doing it. My work as a volunteer for The Neuropathy Association, speaking to people who have called the office for help, helping some people look for a doctor, advising others on how to form a support group, and so on, has been so gratifying. Last spring, I took my own advice: I talked with a friend about starting a new support group. We found a place to meet and have been pleased with our success.

It's amazing. My immune system has been so strengthened by IVIg that I can sit next to anyone who has a cold and I don't catch it.
—Irene Beer

(Now there's the most positive spin on the value of IVIg
I've ever heard. Mims Cushing)

Meet Teri

Teri Turi of Gibraltar is 45, married with four children between the ages of 15 and 20, and works mornings in a children's nursery, five days a week.

Teri echoes what many people with serious peripheral neuropathy have said, that it would be easier if the disability were visible. Peripheral neuropathy is such a "hidden" thing—all the pain and burning cannot be seen by the outside world. For that reason, people with the ailment often feel as if they have to pretend as though nothing is wrong.

Teri relies on a deeper level of spirituality and has become close to fellow PNers, Jan and Judaline; Jan from Illinois helped her raise herself above the negatives of peripheral neuropathy. They talk regularly on the phone. Judaline and Teri met when they were having IVIg. Teri says, "I asked her how she managed to stay so happy. Judaline, who is from South Africa, said she believes everything that happens is part of God's Plan." And Teri gets through the tough days by telling herself that it's all part of the Plan.

A Peripheral Neuropathy Journey from (Almost) Africa to London
By Teri Tura

I am from London, England, currently living in Gibraltar. I belong to the National Peripheral Neuropathy Community (npnc.org).

In 2005, I noticed numbness and tingling in both feet. In the mornings I had no idea of where my feet where. They just felt dead and cold. My podiatrist thought it was a circulation problem. A month later, I felt the same sensations in both hands, then noticed these feelings were traveling symmetrically up my legs and arms. I saw a general practitioner who took blood and found nothing unusual, except that I had no reflexes at all. He suggested Raynaud's syndrome.

As the weather improved, my symptoms worsened. I lost sensation in my right hand, and my left foot and leg became much worse. In 2006, I saw a general neurologist who diagnosed peripheral neuropathy and sent me to Malaga for nerve conduction studies. The results showed no evidence of peripheral neuropathy in my feet, but marked carpal tunnel in both hands, for which I was given wrist splints and offered surgery. The diagnosis upset me because I didn't have pain in my hands, so how could I have a carpal tunnel problem? I declined the surgery.

By this time, the crawling, tingling, numbness had spread to my face and was in patchy areas all over my body. My parents live in London, and they made an appointment with a peripheral neuropathy specialist at the National Hospital for Neurology and Neurosurgery in Central London. In May of 2006, the doctor agreed to take me on as a patient. He ordered blood tests and repeat nerve conduction studies, which showed no evidence of CTS. Over the next few months, I had an MRI [magnetic resonance imaging], a spinal tap, a lip biopsy, and a sural nerve biopsy. The sural nerve is on the side of your foot, and if you have a sural nerve biopsy, that's where it's done. You are permanently numb there following this procedure. The diagnosis was dorsal root ganglionopathy.

Currently I am having regular IVIg treatments in London, and I feel very fortunate to be under the care of my current neurologist.

The hardest part of neuropathy for me is the constancy of it. I used to do yoga, and aerobics, and played tennis, but due to my painful feet and loss of balance, I have had to stop all classes. I swim as much as possible and will try to return to yoga.

I am fortunate in that, so far, only my left foot is affected. Sometimes it feels wet, other times it's as if needles are sticking into it, or that it's being held in a vise. On really bad days, I have wished I could cut it off. Tappings and vibrations are common. I often feel as though I am walking on glass or as though a concrete block is at the end of my leg. Closed shoes are painful, as is walking on a hardwood floor. I feel as if I have lost the fat pads in my feet and am very aware of every stone and pebble.

My right arm feels as though there's a tourniquet above the elbow, and it also feels as though both arms are tightly gripped. My face and neck are constantly crawling, as if cling film covers me and my skin is trying to turn inside out. My back feels as if two fists are pushing into me behind my ribs. Other times it's as if I am wearing a cloak. Meds cause me weight gain and constant fatigue.

I am lucky to have an extremely supportive husband and family, although there was a time when other relatives would ask, "Are you sure you aren't imagining this?"

Sometimes I feel myself slipping into a dark hole, because it is gradually getting worse. Where will I be in 5 or 10 years? I still have awful days and cry. Sometimes I wish my foot was stuck in a bucket of wet cement. Then it would be visible to people and they would be more understanding.

Being an active member of NPNC has been an enormous benefit, as I have gained information, support, and friendship. I am hopeful that one day there will be a cure.

—TERI TURA

Meet Shane

Shane Gibbs' story popped up on my screen one morning. This Australian said he has had neuropathy since he was 6 years old. Neuropathy even catches you if you live down under.

Never Tell Someone They Can't Do Something
By Shane Gibbs

In October of 1969, a gorgeous little kid was born—me! All the body parts were there and in the right places and working as they should ... until around the age of 6. I noticed that I always tripped on my left foot, scraping my toes. My worried mother took me to several doctors who said nothing was wrong and Mum was imagining things. Eventually, a doctor took an interest, sent me to a specialist in Sydney, and started ordering tests.

Before I was 8, I had had several tests. I remember two nerve conduction studies. I am unsure of their names, but I do remember they really hurt. To an 8-year-old having what appeared to be really big needles stuck into him and then zapped with electricity was a big deal. And they did it twice, to test nerves and the muscles. The doctor gave me $10 for being brave. Sadly, I lost the money before we got to the car.

Next came more tests, for which I spent more than a week in a hospital. The tests confirmed I had progressive peripheral neuropathy of the axonal type. What confused the doctors then and still does is that it primarily affects my left foot.

Diets, vitamins, physiotherapy were all to no avail. Helping me walk better was the only thing doctors could do. From the time I first saw the specialist until now, I have worn calipers. I started with the so-called rat-trap calipers. Ugly heavy things, these metal braces permanently attach to solid leather shoes. The idea was to correct a complete foot drop. They had to be replaced often, as I kept outgrowing the shoes. Ever been to school as a kid when there is something different about you? I was teased, bullied, last picked for teams, etc. The world was different then. You ignored things and toughened up.

Somewhere around this time, I was fed up with the calipers. I started wearing light-weight shoes and ignored the foot drop. The doctors decided to try a Grice procedure with "elongation of the tendo-Achillis and probably transferring the tibialis posterior to improve dorsiflexion." (I'm quoting from a medical record.) It meant they would remove my Achilles tendon, attach it to a sliver of bone, which they would remove from the top of my leg, and then join them to my ankle in an effort to keep my foot permanently at right angles. This happened in 1980, when I was 10. I stayed for 2 weeks in the hospital and was on crutches for 3 months. The operation was not a total success. I still had drop foot and still had to wear calipers.

High school was fast approaching. Calipers and high school. Not a pleasant combination. Somewhere around this time, AFOs [ankle-foot orthotics] were developed. These are a form of caliper that's molded to your leg and worn under a sock and any type of shoe. I had a great time smashing the old calipers with a hammer when I first got the AFOs. I spent all my high school years with 90% of the school ignorant of my condition.

In 1983, doctors did further testing at a different hospital so we could get another opinion. They found nothing new. I still had axonal-neuronal neuropathy, and they could not rule out whether it was or wasn't a new mutant variety. Doctors were confused about the asymmetry. The left side was still worse than the right. At that time, only 100 children had my condition, they told me, and I was the second oldest.

At every visit to the doctors they only asked one question: "How much pain are you in?" I can always remember some pain, but I didn't think anything of it. Mum could hear me at night moaning. Today, the pain is pretty much the same. During the day, there's muscular pain either in my arms or legs that feels as though I've been working out. At night, my right leg can get painful. Rubbing and movement are the only cures for this. The interesting symptoms are the electric shocks that shoot up my leg. I first felt them when I was driving. I actually pulled over, thinking I had a loose wire under the dash.

The ground hurts—carpet, grass, sand, etc. Sun, breeze, water are all very uncomfortable. I even swim in jeans. The motion of water around my legs is extremely unpleasant. Jeans seem to mask it. The extra weight of jeans is beneficial in keeping muscle tone in my legs. Unfortunately, the local pool has banned me from swimming because of the jeans. Walking long distances is painful. Sitting in one spot for too long creates leg cramps. My fingers cramp up when I use a keyboard. I have 30% use of the left side of my body, 70% of my right. This hasn't changed in 20 years or so.

All my life, my mother told me I couldn't do this or that. Doctors told me I would never physically be able to do something. Never tell someone that. As a kid, I did all the things a kid did. I rode pushbikes, climbed trees, bush walked, and abseiled, similar to rappelling. I handle snakes—Australia has eight out of ten most deadly species.

I have lost some fitness as I am not riding my bike as much. Twenty years ago, I got a driver's license, then 10 years ago, I added a truck license, and also a motorcycle license. I've worked in retail, driven trucks interstate, climbed on roofs to install pay TV, and more. Currently, I have sole care of my 7-year-old son and do some foster care. I am coping!

I have always had pain somewhere. The difference, and the local GP agrees, is that I am able to block it to a certain degree. Sometimes I could have been screaming blue murder, but I am able to cope, although not always.
—SHANE GIBBS

Meet Terry

Terry Rees lives in the little town of Yreka (pronounced Why-Reeka), in California, 22 miles south of the Oregon border. It sits at the foot of beautiful Mt. Shasta. The winter weather can close roads, sometimes in both directions. Mountains surround the town. If medical attention is needed, it can be a problem with 8–24 inches of snow for three months, which happened in 2008.

Terry, in her mid-60s, co-leads a peripheral neuropathy support group and is part of a small theater troupe. She worked in the field of personnel administration, then in office management, and she owned a print shop and typing service. She has a son and an adopted daughter.

CAUTION: Neuropathy Around the Bend!
By Terry Rees

My first symptoms of neuropathy appeared in 1964 when I was 22 and pregnant with my son. At the time, I assumed the problems were part of my pregnancy. As I look back, I think peripheral neuropathy had a profound effect on my child rearing, as I was tired a good share of the time. I remember feeling insecure when I carried children. When I lifted them, I felt my knees would buckle. My symptoms were (and still are) electrical impulses in my feet, mostly at night, approximately 20 minutes after I have gone to bed. The sensation starts in one leg or the other and feels like a feather is being run down the back of it. Once it reaches the back of my foot, I get a feeling I refer to as being zapped by a cattle prod—an electrical shock in my foot, which makes my foot and sometimes my leg jump. Because of it, I am not able to sleep and must walk around. Although it is not severely painful, it can make me cry.

Over the years, as my symptoms worsened, I would have to get out of bed and walk or sit in a chair until the symptoms stopped, or I until fell asleep, exhausted.

After several hours, the zapping shocks would subside in the affected leg, but would almost immediately start in the other leg, causing me to be up most of the night. This happened more and more, until about 8 years ago my doctor diagnosed my problem: peripheral neuropathy. He put me on medication. I learned to take my pill in the early evening so it would be effective around my bedtime. My husband bought me a watch with an alarm set to 7:00 P.M. and, no matter where I am or what I am doing, when the alarm goes off—at a meeting, on a cruise, in a restaurant—if I'm with friends they will say, "Terry, you are beeping. Take your pill." Sometimes symptoms break through even when I take the pill. Lately, I have begun to have more and more problems, and I believe I am building up an immunity to the meds.

During the day, I would have "hot spots" on my legs. Originally, I suffered from extremely hot feet at night. In the middle of the night I would have to get up and stand in a cool place, such as the bathtub or even out on the lawn, which is difficult to do in the dead of winter with snow on the ground. Oddly, the hot feet have become extremely cold feet. We bought an electric blanket, and I heat the bed before I climb in. When my feet are cold, it takes several hours before they warm up. With the blanket, the warmth penetrates my legs and feet, and it makes all the difference.

A neurologist told me my neuropathy is hereditary, and that my mother and two sisters also have it, having suffered with nerve problems in their knees.

My mother had it for the last 35–40 years of her life. My middle sister recently went through chemo and radiation and has developed neuropathy in her feet as well as her knees.

I also have balance problems, memory problems, and other symptoms, but these are mild and in no way are as intrusive as the problems with my feet. If I get to bed and my feet jump, I still have to get up. Sometimes I get on the computer and play games, which takes my mind off my feet and tires me out more quickly than if I simply walk the floor. If I walk, I get bored and boredom does not necessarily induce sleep. I am not very physically active. A monthly hand and foot massage helps a little.

I have to say the best thing that has happened to me regarding peripheral neuropathy is the formation of our support group. What a great feeling to be among people with the same problems, and what I have learned is amazing. I have formed some wonderful new friendships. I've especially learned that I am not alone.

*Peripheral neuropathy is a difficult thing to live with,
and there isn't a lot of relief out there, but compared to other health
problems, we should consider ourselves lucky. Join or form
a support group. That could help you as much or more
than some prescription medications.*

—TERRY REES

Meet Denise

There's no reason why a person with minimal or even not-so-minimal neuropathy can't travel. It took guts for Denise Weaver, a caregiver and also a volunteer at the Ronald McDonald Room at Wolfson Children's Hospital, Jacksonville, Florida, to go white-water rafting, but she is thrilled she went. She made memories with her family to last forever.

"My Body Was Not Made for This!"
By Denise Weaver

I am 62 years old and have had hereditary neuropathy, with burning and sharp pains in my hands and feet, since my early 40s. My mother and father had the same symptoms, which doctors couldn't diagnose. My peripheral neuropathy has gotten worse through the years, but I have never let it stop me from doing what I want.

Seven adults and four children—a challenge in itself—decided to take a rafting trip on the Nantahala River in North Carolina. It was March, and the temperature was in the 30s. On our first day, we hiked to seven waterfalls. The hardest one was 200 steps down and half a mile up. Going down seemed easy, but I did not think about the climb back up. The view was spectacular, and well worth it; however, my feet and hands were not happy that night.

The next day, we went on a train ride. That was easy, but then the day after that we went white-water rafting in freezing cold water. I put on water-walking shoes and then put my body in a wet suit, which it is not meant for. My feet started out the day cold, and would get a whole lot colder. I got down to my raft and, first thing, fell smack into it, face first. Not a good start. My balance is poor, especially on an unsteady raft. It helped that the guide looked like a young Robert Redford. Three people helped me get onto the right spot, and then it was beautiful and exciting with one rapid after another. I was having too much fun to think about my hands and feet.

Suddenly, we hit a boulder and I was thrown into the ice cold river. What a shocking sensation! They fished me out and flipped me back into the cranky raft. I was soaking wet and freezing. Other than that, the rest of the trip was smooth sailing. My feet were throbbing. Still, it was worth it.

The rest of the week was one adventure after another. Horseback riding, jet boating, hiking.... Every night was a struggle with unusually bad foot pain, but I'd have missed all the fun if I'd stayed behind. I would have been in my typical amount of discomfort at home and missed all the memories.

I will not let this condition rule my life. Keeping busy keeps my mind off it. Exercise is very important. Some days I just say to myself, today's flare-up won't last forever. I am a member of a support group, which has been a lifesaver. Knowing others who are going through this helps. I learn something new every time I go.

Dwelling on your neuropathy does no good. Diverting yourself by traveling is a great way to keep your mind off your peripheral neuropathy.

Taking a trip is a great escape for people with peripheral neuropathy. You may have so much fun you don't have time to think about your feet.
—DENISE WEAVER

The Jacksonville Florida Support Group was saddened to learn that Denise Weaver died in August 2008, at her home. She had been a long-time, valuable member of the group and is missed. At the July meeting, she read her entry for this book, and was elated that it would be published.

Meet Clifford

A few years ago a man named Clifford Meyer introduced himself to a support group in California. He said he'd been a Marine in the Korean War, and gave a few more details, but not enough to satisfy group leader Bev Anderson. She wanted to know what effect the freezing temperatures had on the men while they were in Korea, known to be one of the coldest places on the planet. Meyer and Anderson sat down at a later date, and she recorded his story and transcribed it for this book, with Meyer's permission.

A Korean War Story
As Told to Bev Anderson, by Marine Sgt. Clifford Meyer, USM Ret. One of the "Chosin Few"

Extreme cold can precipitate neuropathy, judging by the experiences of Marines in the 3rd Battalion, 7th Regiment during the Battle of

Chosin Reservoir, Korean War, 1950. The troops were nicknamed the "Chosin Few" or "Frozen Chosin." General Douglas MacArthur was their commander.

About 15,000 troops went into battle. Approximately 8,000 survived. Today, at their reunions, many give evidence of peripheral neuropathy. They fought in subzero weather for weeks. This commonality was increasingly thought to be the cause of their neuropathy.

The 1st Marine Division started out in late September. On November 2, in the region of the Chosin Reservoir, the 2nd Battalion of the 7th Marine Regiment was assaulted by the 124th Regiment of the Chinese Communist People's Army. The battle raged for 3 days. The Marines prevailed, and destroyed most of the Chinese Regiment.

The Chinese disappeared. The Marines thought they went back to Manchuria. The truth is they hid, regrouped, and came out only at night. The bridges over the Yalu River had been bombed, but this was winter and tens of thousands of Chinese troops crossed on solid ice and kept the battle going.

From October to mid-December, the Marines fought in temperatures of –5 degrees Fahrenheit in the daytime and –40 degrees at night. Many men froze to death. All had parkas and helmets, but some had more layers of clothing than others. They had shoe packs made of rubber with a felt insert to absorb the moisture because even in the cold their feet would sweat. If they stopped moving, the sweat would freeze. As they moved around, they were encouraged to keep wiggling their toes. One man reported that he was able to get his boots off and change his socks and felt pads every other day. He'd put the wet pad under one arm to dry and the moist sock he had changed went under the other.

Food was scarce. The Marines put tins with frozen rations under their clothing to thaw them a bit. Gifts that saved their lives were the Tootsie Rolls dropped from supply planes. The men could eat them frozen and not suffer stomach problems. Snow provided their only drinking water because water in the canteens froze. Weapons froze. Blood plasma froze. For the medics, corpsmen carried morphine caps in their mouths to keep the pain killers from freezing. The wounded were covered with canvas or straw and put outside the tents—there were too many men to keep them all inside.

After the Korean War, veterans' organizations formed. In 1983, at meetings, the men talked about strange pains in their feet, legs, and hands. "Pappy" GySgt. Ernest G. Pappenheimer, who lost part of his foot due to the cold, worked to get the Veterans Administra-

*tion [VA] to recognize that the freezing cold had caused the periph-
eral neuropathy, which in turn resulted in amputations. Doctors in
the clinics said the amputations were not needed because of the
cold-induced peripheral neuropathy, but by something else, perhaps
smoking or diabetes.*

*At a reunion in Hawaii, the Secretary of Veterans Affairs, the
Honorable Jesse Brown, listened to the Marines and brought in people from the VA to talk to the vets. As a result, the Marines started
getting disability for their injuries due to the cold.*

*The VA now recognizes the impact that frigid cold had in Korea
and during World War II, and realizes cold can cause peripheral
neuropathy. The VA regularly makes disability pension adjust-
ments because of the impact on the lives of the men who fought in
such extreme conditions.*

*People must take steps to prevent peripheral neuropathy in any
occupation or leisure activity where they are in extreme cold.
People must be made aware of the consequences of long-term
freezing weather.*
—CLIFFORD MEYER

Meet Martha

Martha Chandley, 68, goes well beyond the extra mile when it comes to working as a leader of two neuropathy support groups. The job doesn't have to
involve a tremendous amount of work, but Chandley works tirelessly and
makes beating neuropathy a serious, yet joyful ongoing project. This is her
Mission Statement:

*To be a peripheral neuropathy researcher, writer, publisher,
support group leader, counselor, and advocate before the medical
community, so that no one has to suffer from peripheral neuropathy
alone and all desiring it may be educated, empowered, and
supported in their lives with neuropathy. May we all thrive and
not merely survive with our neuropathy, whatever the cause.*
—MARTHA CHANDLEY

The Healing Power of Helping Others
By Martha Chandley

*In 1998, I was diagnosed with carpal tunnel syndrome [CTS] and
diabetes. The CTS distress and weakness have never totally gone*

away in spite of surgeries on both hands in 1999. The year after that, I began to have typical diabetic peripheral neuropathy symptoms, and was diagnosed in 2001 with a moderate axonal polyneuropathy, presumably from the diabetes, but that was not stated.

I quickly got my diabetes under control by dietary changes, so much so that I was removed from medications. I did water exercises at the YMCA and took antioxidant supplements. My neuropathy symptoms began to recede, but not before I began suffering with continuous burning sensations in my feet and leg. This led to my having to leave work in 2001. I kept myself from going "nuts" by using homeopathic remedies such as transdermal topical Neuragen, Vicks VapoRub, or a wintergreen alcohol/aspirin spray, followed by a thick lotion on my feet when milder symptoms arose.

My most persistent and problematic neuropathic pain has been from spinal stenosis and sciatica, for which a failed partial laminectomy was of little help. Strong pain meds continue to keep me going in the worst times. After suffering two compression spinal fractures in the summer of 2007, I have struggled with extreme neuropathic and other types of pain, exhaustion, and possible fibromyalgia that diminished my functional capacity approximately 65% for months on end. My current medical pain specialist and chiropractor are helping a great deal, but we are far from full resolution and perhaps may never be. Twice-a-week, gentle yoga sessions have also been a great help.

Part of my coping has long centered on reading as much as possible about neuropathy and looking at hundreds of Internet resources. They were and are essential in my helping others with their neuropathy. These resources have also helped me dialog with some of the medical community.

In my early stages of peripheral neuropathy, I became involved with the Sacramento, California, neuropathy support group and served for a time on the board of the Northern California Chapter of The Neuropathy Association (NCCNA), a network of 40 or so groups across our region. I started three support groups in the Woodland, Davis, and West Sacramento communities of Yolo County. All three continue to function with shared leadership.

I publish Peripheral Neuropathy NEWS *monthly, which provides a great deal of information about neuropathy and related health issues for Yolo members and friends, for subscribers in the region, and for people across the U.S.*

In the last year, I've been the 916 area code "Voice" of the NCCNA's Neuropathy Hotline, an ongoing neuropathy public awareness campaign project.

Several times a week, I respond to callers of various income and educational levels, give them counsel on how to get proper diagnostic and treatment services, and encourage them to connect with the nearest support group. If they have no established health care, I send brochures to them regarding public clinics, and urge them to contact the Health Rights Hotline if they have difficulties getting services. They receive an informative "Neuropathy 101" package, developed from a variety of resources, along with brochures about The Neuropathy Association, NCCNA, and specific products. They may also receive condition-specific booklets published by the National Institute for Neurological Disorders and Strokes (NINDS), which they are encouraged to share with their doctors. Newcomers to our support groups receive similar packages of information.

My involvement with The Neuropathy Hotline has made me extremely concerned about the grossly inadequate general health care services for the homeless and other poor suffering with peripheral neuropathy. However inadequate our neuropathy care has been for most of us who are part of America's middle class, it's a thousand times worse for the people I speak with, sometimes daily. I long for the day when all of us middle-class PNers will care enough to advocate for the neuropathy health care needs of the less fortunate and not just our own.

My peripheral neuropathy activism is an integral part of my coping. I thoroughly enjoy my various roles, studying the literature and writing about the issues that impact lives. I care deeply about other people and their struggles with peripheral neuropathy. My plate is full, but if I can get enough restorative rest and pain relief, I'll continue my mission. I marvel at my 89-year-old Dad, grateful that we can live together and care for one another, praising God for sustaining us in our journeys.

My peripheral neuropathy activism is an integral part of my coping.
—MARTHA CHANDLEY

Biographies

If you enjoyed the personal stories included in this book, you may be interested in a 2008 book, *Strong at the Broken Places: Voices of Illness, a Chorus of Hope,* by Richard Cohen,[2] bestselling author and multiple award winner of three Emmys and a Peabody Award. This book features five courageous people battling five illnesses: amyotrophic lateral sclerosis (ALS), Crohn's disease, muscular dystrophy, bipolar disorder, and Hodgkin's lymphoma. Cohen interviewed them over the course of 3 years, to find out how they cope.

Cohen is Meredith Viera's husband. His beautiful memoir about his life with multiple sclerosis made me think about other books by people living with disabilities, whether physical or emotional, and triumphing over adversities. If you enjoy reading this type of book, I've listed a few.

Two books deal directly with neuropathy and are recommended by Dr. Latov and me. One is *Bed Number Ten,* by Sue Baier and Mary Zimmeth Schomaker (CRC Press Inc., 1989).[3] This is a true story of Baier's struggle as she overcomes Guillian-Barre syndrome in an intensive care unit staffed by many careless and noncaring nurses. It is a haunting story of tremendous determination.

Another book on the topic of peripheral neuropathy that we recommend is *Pride and the Daily Marathon,* by Jonathan Cole, MD,[4] a clinical neurophysiologist at Poole Hospital, Cambridge, England. Cole writes the story of Ian Waterman, whose rare form of peripheral neuropathy struck him at age 19. He learned to compensate for his sensory neuropathy and total lack of sensation—the worst case his medical consultant had ever seen. The famed author Oliver Sachs thought the story to be "at once terrifying and inspiring ... a neurological epic."

Sitting on my bookshelves, I found a couple dozen of memoirs I've especially loved, most of which I reviewed for the *Florida Times-Union* in the 1990s. These are listed in the For Further Reading section.[1-28] They, too, are stories of people struggling and triumphing despite difficult issues. Read them when you are having a tough time, or not.

For Further Reading

1. Senneff, John A. *Numb Toes and Aching Soles: Coping with Peripheral Neuropathy.* San Antonio: MedPress, 1999.

2. Cohen, Richard. *Strong at the Broken Places: Voices of Illness, a Chorus of Hope.* New York: Harper, 2008.

3. Baier, Sue, and Mary Zimmeth Schomaker. *Bed Number Ten.* Boca Raton, FL: CRC Press Inc., 1989.

4. Cole, Jonathan. *Pride and the Daily Marathon,* Cambridge: MIT Press, 1995.

5. Ashworth, Andrea. *Once in a House on Fire.* New York: Henry Holt, 1998.

6. Balakian, Peter. *Black Dog of Fate.* New York: Broadway Books, 1997.

7. Beck, Martha. *Expecting Adam.* New York: Times Books/Random House, 1997.

8. Black, Kathryn. *In the Shadow of Polio: A Personal and Social History*. New York: Addison-Wesley, 1996.

9. Cohen, Richard M. *Blindsided: Living a Life Above Illness*. New York: Harper-Collins, 2004.

10. Cutting, Linda Katherine. *Memory Slips: A Memoir of Music and Healing*. New York: Harper Perennial, 1997.

11. Davidson, Ann. *Alzheimer's, A Love Story: One Year in My Husband's Journey*. Secaus, NJ: Carol Publishing Group, 1997.

12. Dominick, Andie. *Needles: A Memoir of Growing Up with Diabetes*. New York: Scribner, 1998.

13. Finneran, Kathleen. *The Tender Land: A Family Love Story*. New York: Houghton Mifflin, 2000.

14. Fraizer, Ian. *Family*. New York: Farrar Straus Giroux, 1994.

15. French, Marilyn. *A Season in Hell*. New York: Knopf, 1998.

16. Harrison, Barabara Grizzuti. *An Accidental Autobiography*. New York: Houghton Mifflin, 1996.

17. Jamison, Kay Redfield. *An Unquiet Mind: A Memoir of Moods and Madness*. New York: Vintage Books/Random House, 1995.

18. Lauck, Jennifer. *Blackbird: A Childhood Lost and Found*. New York: Washington Square Press, 2000.

19. Lessing, Doris. *Under My Skin: Volume One of My Autobiography, to 1949*. New York: Harper Perennial, 1994.

20. McCrum, Robert. *My Year Off: Recovering Life After a Stroke*. New York: W.W. Norton, 1998.

21. Middlebrook, Christina. *Seeing the Crab: A Memoir of Dying Before I Do*. New York: Anchor Books/Doubleday, 1996.

22. Radner, Gilda. *It's Always Something*. New York: Simon and Schuster, 1989.

23. Rhett, Kathryn, ed. *Survival Stories: Memoirs of Crisis*. New York: Doubleday, 1997.

24. Sexton, Linda Gray. *Searching for Mercy Street*. New York: Little, Brown and Company, 1994.

25. Shapiro, Dani. *Slow Motion*. New York: Random House, 1998.

26. Slater, Lauren. *Welcome to My Country*. New York: Random House, 1999.

27. Synder, Don J. *Of Time and Memory: A Mother's Story*. New York: Knopf, 1999.

28. Zabbia, Kim Howes. *Painted Diaries: A Mother and Daughter's Experience Through Alzheimer's*. Minneapolis, MN: Fairview Press, 1996.

The Neuropathy Association's Designated Neuropathy Centers

To learn more about the designated neuropathy centers in the United States, check with The Neuropathy Association at 800-247-6968 to find one near you. These institutes offer

- Sophisticated evaluation, diagnoses, and treatment by physicians specifically trained in neuromuscular disease
- A systematic approach to classify peripheral neuropathy based on clinical features, identification of the type of nerve fiber involved, the distribution or pattern of nerve fiber involvement, and the mode of evolution (acute, subacute, or chronic)
- State-of-the-art neurophysiologic assessment including nerve conduction/electromyographic (EMG) studies, single-fiber EMG quantitative threshold determinations, quantitative motor testing, and tremor analysis
- Neuropathologic assessment of nerve and muscle biopsies
- Pioneering research

Resources

Some of these groups will send you, free, a brochure or information about their organization.

American Academy of Medical Acupuncture
4929 Wilshire Boulevard, Ste. 428
Los Angeles, CA 90036
800-521-2262
www.medicalacupuncture.org

American Academy of Neurology
1080 Montreal Avenue
St. Paul, MN 55116
800-879-1960
www.aan.com

American Academy of Orthopedic Surgeons
630 North River Road
Rosemont, IL 60018
800-346-AAOS
www.aaos.org

American Academy of Pain Medicine
4700 West Lake Avenue
Glenview, IL 60025
847-375-4731
info@painmed.org
www.painmed.org

American Board of Hypnotherapy
16842 Von Karman Avenue, Suite 475
Irvine, CA 92606
800-872-9996
www.hypnosis.com

American Chronic Pain Association
P.O. Box 850
Rocklin, CA 95677
800-533-3231
www.theacpa.org

American Diabetes Association
1701 North Beauregard Street
Alexandria, VA 22311
800-342-2383
askade@diabetes.org
www.diabetes.org

American Holistic Health Association
P.O. Box 17400
Anaheim, CA 92817-7400
714-779-6152
mail@ahha.org
www.ahha.org

American Massage Therapy Association
500 Davis Street, Ste. 900
Evanston, IL 60201-4695
847-864-0123
www.amtamassage.org

American Orthopaedic Foot and Ankle Society
6300 North River Road, Ste. 510
Rosemont, IL 60018
800-235-4855
www.aofas.org

American Pain Society
4700 West Lake Avenue
Glenview, IL 60025-1485
847-375-4715
www.ampainsoc.org

American Pain Foundation
888-615-7246
www.painfoundation.org.

Anodyne Therapy
13570 Wright Circle
Tampa, FL 33626
800-521-6664
www.anodynetherapy.com

The Association for Driver Rehabilitation Specialists
877-529-1830
www.aded.net

Center for Psychological and Spiritual Health
www.cpsh.org.

Charcot Marie Tooth Association
2700 Chestnut Street
Chester, PA 19013
800-606-CMTA (2682)
www.charcot-marie-tooth.org

Complementary Alternative Medicine Association
cama@camaweb.org
www.camaweb.org

Florida Chapter Neuropathy Support Network
Nine Lecture/Discussions available free by e-mail or for postage by regular
mail. Reviewed by two neuromuscular neurologists and written by a patient
with peripheral neuropathy.
954-328-1630
prcgene@aol.com

GBS/CIDP Foundation International
The Holly Building
104½ Forrest Avenue
Narbeth, PA 19072
866-224-3301
info@gb-cidp.org
www.gbs-cidp.org

Hay House
Tapes for meditating
Box 5100
Carlsbad, CA 90218-5100
800-654-5126
www.hayhouse.com

Hereditary Neuropathy Foundation
1751 Second Avenue, Ste. 103
New York NY 10128
877-463-1287; 212-722-8396
info@hnf-cure.org
www.hnf-cure.org

International Association of Mind-Body Professionals
30245 Tomas
Rancho Santa Margarita, CA 92688
949-589-9166
www.mind-bodypro.com

International Institute of Reflexology
P.O. Box 12642
St. Petersburg, FL 33733
813-343-4811
www.reflexology.org

Jack Miller Center for Peripheral Neuropathy
http://millercenter.uchicago.edu/index.shtml

Kids Health Organization
How to deal with the medical and emotional impact of caring for an ill child
www.kidshealth.org/parent/system/ill/seriouslyill.html.

Kripalu Center for Yoga and Health
P.O. Box 309
Stockbridge MA 01262
413-448-3400
www.kripalu.org.

National Institute of Neurological Disorders and Stroke
800-352-9424
www.ninds.nih.gov

National Mobility Equipment Dealers Association
3327 West Bearss Avenue
Tampa, FL 33618
800-833-0427
www.nmeda.org

National Pain Foundation
www.nationalpainfoundation.org

The Neuropathy Association
60 East 42nd Street, Ste. 942
New York, NY 10165
800-247-6968
www.neuropathy.org

NORD (Nat'l Organization of Rare Diseases)
55 Kenosia Avenue
Danbury, CT 06810
203-744-0100
www.rarediseases.org

Northern California Chapter of The Neuropathy Association
916-371-1125
www.pnhelp.org
www.neuropathy.org

Patient Advocate Foundation
www.patientadvocate.org

Patient Services Incorporated
Co-payment waiver assistance for people with chronic illnesses
800-366-7741
www.uneedpsi.org

Sjögren's Syndrome Foundation
6707 Democracy Boulevard
Bethesda MD 20817
800-475-6473
www. sjogrens.org

Wheelchair Foundation
3820 Blackhawk Road
Danville, CA 94506-4617
925-791-2340
www.wheelchairfoundaton.org

World Research Foundation
The Foundation will send you hundreds of pages relating to your neuropathy or other medical problem. It has a 25,000-book library. There is a charge for the service.
928-284-3300
www.wrf.org

Acronyms

CIDP	Chronic inflammatory demyelinating polyneuropathy
CMT	Charcot-Marie-Tooth. A hereditary neuropathy named after three doctors
CTS	Carpal tunnel syndrome. An entrapment neuropathy
DPN	Diabetic peripheral neuropathy
EMG	Electromyography. A diagnostic test
GBS	Guillain-Barré syndrome
IVIg	Intravenous immunoglobulin (sometimes seen as intravenous gamma globulin)
NCCNA	Northern California Chapter of The Neuropathy Association
NINDS	National Institute for Neurological Disorders and Strokes
NPNC	National Peripheral Neuropathy Community
PNers	People who have peripheral neuropathy
QST	Quantitative sensory testing
TNA	The Neuropathy Association

Bibliography

Ashworth, Andrea. *Once in a House on Fire*. New York: Henry Holt, 1998.

Baier, Sue, and Mary Zimmeth Schomaker. *Bed Number Ten*. Boca Raton, FL: CRC Press Inc., 1989.

Bailey, Simon T. *Release Your Brilliance*. New York: HarperCollins, 2008.

Beck, Martha. *Expecting Adam*. New York: Times Books/Random House, 1997.

Bender, Sue. *Plain and Simple: A Woman's Journey to the Amish*. New York: Harper & Row, 1989.

Bersky, Arthur, and Emily C. Deans. *Stop Being Your Symptoms Start Being Yourself. A Six Week Mind-Body Program to Ease Your Chronic Symptoms*. New York: HarperCollins, 2006.

Biebel, David B., and Harold G. Koenig. *New Light on Depression*. Grand Rapids: Zondervan, 2004.

Black, Kathryn. *In the Shadow of Polio: A Personal and Social History*. New York: Addison-Wesley, 1996.

Bolen, Jean Shinoda. *Close to the Bone: Life-Threatening Illness and the Search for Meaning*. New York: Touchstone, 1996.

Bowden, Jonny. *The Most Effective Natural Cures on Earth*. Beverly MA: Fair Winds Press, 2008.

Breathnach, Sarah Ban. *The Simple Abundance Journal of Gratitude*. New York: Warner Books, 1996.

Byrne, Robert. *The 2,548 Best Things Anybody Ever Said*. New York: Galahad Books, a Division of BBS Publishing Corporation, 1996.

Callone, Patricia, and Connie Kudlacek, Barbara C., Vasiloff, Janaan Manternach, and Roger Brumback. *Alzheimer's Disease: 300 Tips for Making Life Easier*. New York: Demos Medical Publishing, 2006.

Carlson, Richard. *You Can Be Happy No Matter What: 4 Principles Your Therapist Never Told You*. San Rafael: New World Library, 1992.

Chopra, Depak. *The Path to Love: Renewing the Power of Spirit in Your Life*. New York: Harmony Books, a division of Crown Publishers, 1997.

Cohen, Richard M. *Strong at the Broken Places: Voices of Illness, a Chorus of Hope.* New York: HarperCollins, 2008.

Cohen, Richard M. *Blindsided: Lifting a Life Above Illness A Reluctant Memoir.* New York: HarperCollins, 2004.

Cole, Jonathan. *Pride and the Daily Marathon.* Cambridge: MIT Press, 1995.

Conari Press Editors. *More Random Acts of Kindness.* Berkeley: Conari Press, 1994.

Conari Press Editors. *Random Acts of Kindness.* Berkeley: Conari Press, 1993.

Connellan, Thomas K. *Bringing Out the Best in Others.* Austin: Bard Press. 2003.

Cooke, Margaret, with Elizabeth Putnan. *Ways You Can Help: Creative, Practical Suggestions for Family and Friends of Patients and Caregivers.* New York: Warner Books, 1996.

Cowles, Jane. *Pain Relief: How to Say No to Acute, Chronic, & Cancer Pain!* New York: Mastermedia Limited, 1993.

Cros, Didier. *Peripheral Neuropathy: A Practical Approach to Diagnosis and Management.* Philadelphia: Lippincott Williams & Wilkins, 2001.

Cutting, Linda Katherine. *Memory Slips: A Memoir of Music and Healing.* New York: Harper Perennial, 1997.

Davidson, Ann. *Alzheimer's: A Love Story One Year in My Husband's Journey.* Carol Publishing Group, 1997.

Dillard, James, and Terra Ziporyn. *Alternative Medicine for Dummies.* Foster City: IDG Books, 1998.

Dominick, Andie. *Needles: A Memoir of Growing Up with Diabetes.* New York: Scribner, 1998.

Donoghue, Paul J., and Mary Siegel. *Living with Invisible Chronic Illness: Sick and Tired of Being Sick and Tired.* New York: Norton, 1992.

Dossey, Larry. *The Extraordinary Healing Power of Ordinary Things: Fourteen Natural Steps to Health and Happiness.* New York: Harmony, 2006.

Edwards, Paul and Sarah. *Working from Home: Everything You Need to Know about Living and Working Under the Same Roof.* New York: Jeffrey Tarcher/Putnam, 1999.

Egoscue, Peter, with Roger Gittines. *Pain Free: A Revolutionary Method for Stopping Chronic Pain.* New York: Bantam Books, 2000.

Finneran, Kathleen. *The Tender Land: A Family Love Story.* New York: Houghton Mifflin, 2000.

Flora, Elizabeth. *Making Friends with Pain.* St. Louis: Sadie Books, 1999.

French, Marilyn. *A Season in Hell.* New York: Knopf, 1998.

Fulghum, Debra Bruce, Bruce Harris McIlwain, and Joel C. Silverfield. *Winning with Chronic Illness: A Complete Program for Health and Well-Being.* Amherst: Prometheus, 1994.

Germer, Fawn. *Hard Won Wisdom.* New York: A Perigee Book, division of Berkley Publishing Group, 2001.

Goldberg, Bonni, and Geo Kendall. *Gifts from the Heart.* Chicago: Contemporary Books, 1990.

Goldstsein, Mel, and Dave Tanner. *Swimming Past 50.* Champaign, IL: Human Kinetics, 1999.

Goleman, Daniel, and Joel Gurin. *Mind Body Medicine: How to Use Your Mind for Better Health*. Yonkers: Consumer Reports Books, 1993.

Gray, John. *Why Mars and Venus Collide: Improving Relationships by Understanding How Men and Women Cope Differently with Stress*. New York: HarperCollins. 2008.

Groopman, Jerome. *The Anatomy of Hope: How People Prevail in the Face of Illness*. New York: Random House, 2004.

Groopman, Jerome. *How Doctors Think*. New York: Houghton Mifflin, 2007.

Halpern, Susan P. *The Etiquette of Illness: What to Say When You Can't Find the Words*. New York: Bloomsbury, 2004.

Hanby-Robie, Sharon. *Simple Friendships: The Spirit of Simple Living*. Carmel, NY: Guideposts, 2005.

Harrington, Anne. *The Cure Within: A History of Mind-Body Medicine*. New York: W.W. Norton, 2008.

Harrison, Barabara Grizzuti. *An Accidental Autobiography*. New York: Houghton Mifflin, 1996.

Hart, Archibald, and Catherine Hart Weber. *Unveiling Depression in Women: A Practical Guide to Understanding and Overcoming Depression*. Grand Rapids: Fleming H. Revell, 2002.

Hill, Beth Ann. *Multiple Sclerosis*: New York: Avery/Penguin Group, 2003.

Hoffman, Donald L. *How to Talk with Your Doctor*. Laguna Beach: Basic Health Publications, 2006.

Hutton, Cleo. *After a Stroke: 300 Tips for Making Life Easier*. New York: Demos Medical Publishing, 2005.

Jacobs, Pamela D. *500 Tips for Coping with Chronic Illness*. San Francisco: Robert D. Reed Publishers, 1995.

Joffe, Rosalind, and Joan Friedlander. *Women, Work, and Autoimmune Disease*. New York: Demos Medical Publishing, 2008.

Keckley, Paul. *99 Questions You Should Ask Your Doctor and Why*. Nashville: Rutledge Hill Press, 1994.

Keene, Nancy. *Working with Your Doctor: Getting the Healthcare You Deserve*. Sebastopol, CA: O'Reilly & Associates, 1998.

Kipfer, Barbara Ann. *14,000 Things to Be Happy about*. New York: Workman, 1990.

Klauser, Henriette Anne. *Put Your Heart on Paper: Staying Connected in a Loose-Ends World*. New York: Bantam Books, 1995.

Kunz, Barbara and Kevin. *Complete Reflexology for Life*. London: DK Adult, 2007.

Latov, Norman. *Peripheral Neuropathy: When the Numbness, Weakness, and Pain Won't Stop A Guide for Patients and Their Families*. New York: American Academy of Neurology/Demos Medical Publishing, 2007.

Lauck, Jennifer. *Blackbird: A Childhood Lost and Found*. New York: Washington Square Press, 2000.

Layard, Richard. *Happiness: Lessons from a New Science*. New York: The Penguin Group, 2005.

Lessing, Doris. *Under My Skin Volume One of My Autobiography, to 1949*. New York: Harper Perennial, 1994.

Levine, Suzanne M. *50 Ways to Ease Foot Pain.* Lincolnwood, IL: Publications International, 1994.

Lipsyte, Robert. *In the Country of Illness: Comfort and Advice for the Journey.* New York: Alfred A. Knopf, 1998.

Lorig, Kate Halsted Holman, David Sobel, Diana Laurent, Virginia Gonzalez, and Marian Minor. *Living a Healthy Life with Chronic Conditions.* Palo Alto: Bull Publishing Company, 2003.

Lucado, Max. *Cure for the Common Life: Living in Your Sweet Spot.* Nashville: W Publishing Group, 2005.

Martin, Paul. *The Healing Mind.* New York: A Thomas Dunne book, an imprint of St. Martin's Press, 1997.

McCrum, Robert. *My Year Off: Recovering Life After a Stroke.* New York: W.W. Norton & Company, Inc., 1998.

Middlebrook, Christina. *Seeing the Crab: A Memoir of Dying Before I Do.* New York: Anchor Books/Doubleday, 1996.

Moyers, Bill. *Healing and the Mind.* New York: Doubleday, 1993.

Myss, Caroline. *Anatomy of the Spirit: The Seven Stages of Power and Healing.* New York: Harmony Books, 1996.

Myss, Caroline. *Why People Don't Heal and How They Can.* New York: Harmony Books, 1997.

Nakazawa, Donna Jackson. T*he Autoimmune Epidemic: Bodies Gone Haywire in a World out of Balance and the Cutting-Edge Science That Promises Hope.* New York: Touchstone, 2008.

O'Hara, Dorene. *Heal the Pain, Comfort the Spirit: The Hows and Whys of Modern Pain Treatment.* Philadelphia: University of Pennsylvania Press, 2002.

Orloff, Judith. *Dr. Judith Orloff's Guide to Intuitive Healing.* New York: Times Books, a division of Random House, 2000.

Orloff, Judith. *Positive Energy: 10 Extraordinary Prescriptions for Transforming Fatigue, Stress, & Fear into Vibrance, Strength, & Love.* New York: Harmony Books, a member of Crown Publishing Group, Division of Random House, 2004.

Parker, Steve. *The Human Body Book.* New York: DK, 2007.

Pausch, Randy. *The Last Lecture.* New York: Hyperion, 2008.

Pelzer, Dave. *Help Yourself: Celebrating the Rewards of Resilience and Gratitude.* New York: Penguin Putnam, Inc., 2000.

Peterson, Melody. *Our Daily Meds: How Pharmaceutical Companies Transformed Themselves into Slick Marketing Machines and Hooked the Nation on Prescription Drugs.* New York: Sarah Crichton Books/Farrar, Straus and Giroux, 2008.

Pizzorno, Joseph. *Total Wellness: Discover the Body's Healing Systems and How They Work For You.* Rocklin: Prima Health, a Division of Prima Publishing, 1998.

Progoff, Ira. *At a Journal Workshop: The Basic Text and Guide for Using the Intensive Journal.* New York: Dialogue House Library, 1975.

Radner, Gilda. *It's Always Something.* New York: Simon and Schuster, 1989.

Ratey, John J. *Spark: The Revolutionary New Science of Exercise and the Brain.* New York: Little, Brown & Company, 2008.

Remen, Rachel Naomi. *My Grandfather's Blessings: Stories of Strength, Refuge, and Belonging*. New York: Riverhead Trade, 2001.

Remen, Rachel Naomi. *Kitchen Table Wisdom: Stories That Heal*. New York: Riverhead Books, 1996.

Rhett, Kathryn, ed. *Survival Stories: Memoirs of Crisis*. New York: Doubleday, 1997.

Roizen, Michael F., and Mehmet C. Oz. *YOU: The Smart Patient: The Insider's Handbook for Getting the Best Treatment*. New York: Free Press. 2006.

Roizen, Michael F. and Mehmet C. Oz. *YOU: Staying Young: The Owner's Manual for Extending Your Warranty*. New York: Free Press, 2007.

Rosenfeld, Arthur. *The Truth about Chronic Pain*. New York: Basic Books, 2003.

Rubin, Alan. *Diabetes for Dummies*. Indianapolis: Wiley Publishing, Inc., 2004.

Schwartz, Shelley Peterman. *Parkinson's Disease: 300 Tips for Making Life Easier*. New York. Demos Medical Publishing, 2006.

Seneff, John A. *Numb Toes and Aching Soles: Coping with Peripheral Neuropathy*. San Antonio, TX: MedPress, 1999.

Senneff, John A. *Numb Toes and Other Woes: More on Peripheral Neuropathy*. San Antonio: MedPress, 2001.

Sexton, Linda Gray. *Searching for Mercy Street*. New York: Little, Brown and Company, 1994.

Shapiro, Dani. *Slow Motion*. New York: Random House, 1998.

Shields, David. *The Thing about Life Is That One Day You'll Be Dead*. New York: Alfred A. Knopf, 2008.

Showker, Kay, with Bob Sehlinger. *The Unofficial Guide to Cruises: Lines & Ships Ranked & Rated, Best Cruise Deals*. New York: John Wiley & Sons, 2007.

Siegel, Bernie S. Love, *Medicine and Miracles: Lessons Learned about Self-Healing from a Surgeon's Experience with Exceptional Patients*. New York: Harper Perennial, 1990.

Sierpina, Victor. *100 Cures for 200 Ailments: Integrated Alternative and Conventional Treatments for the Most Common Illnesses*. New York: Collins, an Imprint of HarperCollins, 2008.

Slater, Lauren. *Welcome to My Country*. New York: Random House, 1999.

Stoddard, Alexandra. *Choosing Happiness: Keys to a Joyful Life*. New York: HarperCollins, 2002.

Stoddard, Alexandra. *Gracious Living in a New World: Finding Joy in Changing Times*. New York: William Morrow and Company: 1996.

Swanson, David W., Editor-in-Chief. *Mayo Clinic on Chronic Pain*. Rochester, MN: The Mayo Foundation, 1999.

Swartzberg, John Edward, and Sheldon Margen. *The Complete Home Wellness Handbook*. New York: Rebus, 2001.

Synder, Don J. *Of Time and Memory: A Mother's Story*. New York: Knopf, 1999.

Tracanelli, Carina. *The Complete Book of Home Crafts: Projects for Adventurous Beginners*. London: New Burlington Books, 2000.

Tsalaky, Teresa. *To Life: A Guide to Finding Your Path Back to Health*. Crescent City, CA: To Life Publications, 2002.

Vonhof, John. *Fixing Your Feet: Preventative Maintenance and Treatment for Foot Problem of Runners, Hikers, and Adventure Racers.* Enumclaw, WA: WinePress Publications, 1997.

Walsh, Peter. *Does This Clutter Make My Butt Look Fat?* New York: Free Press, a division of Simon & Schuster, 2008.

Walsh, Peter. *It's All Too Much: An Easy Plan for Living a Richer Life with Less Stuff.* New York: Free Press, a division of Simon & Schuster, 2006

Weaver, Frances. *I'm Not As Old As I Used to Be: Reclaiming your Life in the Second Half.* New York: Hyperion, 1997.

Weill, Andrew. *8 Weeks to Optimum Health.* New York: Alfred A. Knopf, 1997.

Weiner, Eric. *The Geography of Bliss.* New York: Twelve/Hachette Book Group USA, 2008.

Yoakum, Robert H. *Restless Legs Syndrome: Relief and Hope for Sleepless Victims of a Hidden Epidemic.* New York: Fireside Books/ Simon and Schuster, 2006.

Zabbia, Kim Howes. *Painted Diaries: A Mother and Daughter's Experience Through Alzheimer's.* Minneapolis, MN: Fairview Press, 1996.

Index